Ruminant Diagnostics and Interpretation

Editors

JOHN DUSTIN LOY
JESSIE D. MONDAY
DAVID R. SMITH

VETERINARY CLINICS OF NORTH AMERICA: FOOD ANIMAL PRACTICE

www.vetfood.theclinics.com

Consulting Editor
ROBERT A. SMITH

March 2023 • Volume 39 • Number 1

ELSEVIER

1600 John F. Kennedy Boulevard • Suite 1800 • Philadelphia, Pennsylvania, 19103-2899

http://www.vetfood.theclinics.com

VETERINARY CLINICS OF NORTH AMERICA: FOOD ANIMAL PRACTICE Volume 39, Number 1
March 2023 ISSN 0749-0720, ISBN-13: 978-0-323-93837-2

Editor: Taylor Hayes
Developmental Editor: Axell Ivan Jade M. Purificacion

Veterinary Clinics of North America: Food Animal Practice (ISSN 0749-0720) is published in March, July, and November by Elsevier Inc., 360 Park Avenue South, New York, NY 10010-1710. Subscription prices are $267.00 per year (domestic individuals), $533.00 per year (domestic institutions), $100.00 per year (domestic students/residents), $289.00 per year (Canadian individuals), $702.00 per year (Canadian institutions), $342.00 per year (international individuals), $702.00 per year (international institutions), $100.00 per year (Canadian students), and $165.00 (international students). To receive student/resident rate, orders must be accompanied by name of affiliated institution, date of term, and the signature of program/residency coordinator on institution letterhead. *Clinics* subscription prices. All prices are subject to change without notice. **POSTMASTER:** Send address changes to *Veterinary Clinics of North America: Food Animal Practice*, Elsevier Health Sciences Division, Subscription Customer Service, 3251 Riverport Lane, Maryland Heights, MO 63043. Customer Service (orders, claims, online, change of address): Elsevier Health Sciences Division, Subscription **Customer Service, 3251 Riverport Lane, Maryland Heights, MO 63043. Tel: 1-800-654-2452 (U.S. and Canada); 314-447-8871 (ouside U.S. and Canada). Fax: 314-447-8029. E-mail: journalscustomerservice-usa@elsevier.com (for print support); journalsonlinesupport-usa@elsevier.com (for online support).**

Reprints. For copies of 100 or more, of articles in this publication, please contact the Commercial Reprints Department, Elsevier Inc., 360 Park Avenue South, New York, NY 10010-1710. Tel.: 212-633-3874; Fax: 212-633-3820; E-mail: reprints@elsevier.com.

Veterinary Clinics of North America: Food Animal Practice is covered in *Current Contents/Agriculture, Biology and Environmental Sciences, MEDLINE/PubMed (Index Medicus), and Excerpta Medica.*

Contributors

CONSULTING EDITOR

ROBERT A. SMITH, DVM, MS
Diplomate, American Board of Veterinary Practitioners, Veterinary Research and Consulting Services, LLC, Greeley, Colorado; Veterinary Research and Consulting Services, LLC, Stillwater, Oklahoma, USA

EDITORS

JOHN DUSTIN LOY, DVM, PhD
Diplomate, American College of Veterinary Microbiologists, Professor and Veterinary Microbiologist, Nebraska Veterinary Diagnostic Center, School of Veterinary Medicine and Biomedical Sciences, University of Nebraska-Lincoln, Lincoln, Nebraska, USA

JESSIE D. MONDAY, DVM, MS
Diplomate, American College of Veterinary Preventive Medicine, Bovine Veterinary Diagnostician, Texas A&M Veterinary Medical Diagnostic Laboratory, Canyon, Canyon, Texas, USA

DAVID R. SMITH, DVM, PhD
Diplomate, American College of Veterinary Preventive Medicine, Diplomate, Epidemiology Specialty, Professor and Associate Dean of Research and Graduate Studies, College of Veterinary Medicine, Mississippi State University, Mississippi State, Mississippi, USA

AUTHORS

PAMELA R.F. ADKINS, DVM, PhD
Diplomate, American College of Veterinary Internal Medicine (Large Animal Internal Medicine), Assistant Professor, Department of Veterinary Medicine and Surgery, College of Veterinary Medicine, University of Missouri, Columbia, Missouri, USA

JUAN CARLOS ARANGO-SABOGAL, DMV, PhD
Département de Pathologie et Microbiologie, Faculté de Médecine Vétérinaire, Université de Montréal, St-Hyacinthe, Québec, Canada

BRUCE W. BRODERSEN, DVM, PhD
Professor and Director, Nebraska Veterinary Diagnostic Center, School of Veterinary Medicine and Biomedical Sciences, University of Nebraska-Lincoln, Lincoln, Nebraska, USA

SÉBASTIEN BUCZINSKI, DR VÉT, MSC
Département des Sciences Cliniques, Faculté de Médecine Vétérinaire, Université de Montréal, St-Hyacinthe, Québec, Canada

MICHAEL L. CLAWSON, PhD
Research Molecular Biologist, USDA, Agriculture Research Service, US Meat Animal Research Center, Clay Center, Nebraska, USA

SIMON DUFOUR, DMV, PhD
Département de Pathologie et Microbiologie, Faculté de Médecine Vétérinaire, Université de Montréal, St-Hyacinthe, Québec, Canada

VIRGINIA R. FAJT, DVM, PhD
Diplomate, American College of Veterinary Clinical Pharmacology; Clinical Professor, Veterinary Physiology and Pharmacology, Texas A&M University, College Station, Texas, USA

MATTHEW M. HILLE, DVM, PhD
Assistant Professor and Diagnostic Pathologist, Nebraska Veterinary Diagnostic Center, School of Veterinary Medicine and Biomedical Sciences, University of Nebraska-Lincoln, Lincoln, Nebraska, USA

JOHN DUSTIN LOY, DVM, PhD
Diplomate, American College of Veterinary Microbiologists, Professor and Veterinary Microbiologist, Nebraska Veterinary Diagnostic Center, School of Veterinary Medicine and Biomedical Sciences, University of Nebraska-Lincoln, Lincoln, Nebraska, USA

BRIAN V. LUBBERS, DVM, PhD
Diplomate, American College of Veterinary Clinical Pharmacology; Associate Professor, Food Animal Therapeutics-Outreach, Kansas State University, Manhattan, Kansas, USA

JOHN R. MIDDLETON, DVM, PhD
Diplomate, American College of Veterinary Internal Medicine (Large Animal Internal Medicine), Professor, Department of Veterinary Medicine and Surgery, College of Veterinary Medicine, University of Missouri, Columbia, Missouri, USA

JESSIE D. MONDAY, DVM, MS
Diplomate, American College of Veterinary Preventive Medicine, Bovine Veterinary Diagnostician, Texas A&M Veterinary Medical Diagnostic Laboratory–Canyon, Canyon, Texas, USA

ELIZABETH PARKER, BVSc, MPH, PhD, DACVPM
Dipl ACVPM, Dipl Epidemiology, Department of Veterinary Preventive Medicine, The Ohio State University, Columbus, Ohio, USA

SARAH J. SILLMAN, DVM, PhD
Diplomate American College of Veterinary Pathologists; Assistant Professor and Diagnostic Pathologist, Nebraska Veterinary Diagnostic Center, School of Veterinary Medicine and Biomedical Sciences, University of Nebraska-Lincoln, Lincoln, Nebraska, USA

DAVID R. SMITH, DVM, PhD
Diplomate, American College of Veterinary Preventive Medicine, Diplomate of Epidemiology, Professor and Associate Dean for Research and Graduate Studies, College of Veterinary Medicine, Mississippi State University, Mississippi State, Mississippi, USA

ROBERT J. VAN SAUN, DVM, MS, PhD
Diplomate, American College of Theriogenologists, Diplomate, American College of Veterinary Internal Medicine (Nutrition specialty), Professor and Extension Veterinarian,

Department of Veterinary and Biomedical Sciences, College of Agricultural Sciences, Pennsylvania State University, University Park, Pennsylvania, USA

LEYI WANG, DVM, PhD
Diplomate of the American College of Veterinary Microbiology (DACVM), Clinical Assistant Professor, Department of Veterinary Clinical Medicine, Veterinary Diagnostic Laboratory, College of Veterinary Medicine, University of Illinois at Urbana-Champaign, Urbana, Illinois, USA

YVONNE M. WIKANDER, DVM, MS
Diplomate, American College of Veterinary Pathologists, Clinical Assistant Professor of Veterinary Clinical Pathology, Department of Veterinary Pathobiology, VERO Program, Texas A&M, School of Veterinary Medicine, Canyon, Texas, USA

REBECCA P. WILKES, DVM, PhD
Diplomate of the American College of Veterinary Microbiology (DACVM) (Virology and Bacteriology/Mycology), Associate Professor, Department of Comparative Pathobiology and Molecular Section Head, Animal Disease Diagnostic Laboratory, Purdue University College of Veterinary Medicine, West Lafayette, Indiana, USA

CHRISTINA WILSON-FRANK, MS, PhD
Clinical Associate Professor of Toxicology, Indiana Animal Disease Diagnostic Laboratory, Department of Comparative Pathobiology, Clinical Associate Professor of Toxicology and Head, Analytical Chemist, Purdue University College of Veterinary Medicine, West Lafayette, Indiana, USA

AMELIA R. WOOLUMS, DVM, MVSc, PhD
Mikell and Mary Cheek Hall Davis Endowed Professor, Department of Pathobiology and Population Medicine, Mississippi State University, Mississippi State, Mississippi, USA

Contents

> Diagnostic tests are performed daily by bovine practitioners at the individual and population level. At the individual level, they help not only for making a diagnosis, but can also serve to rule in or rule out a specific condition, monitor treatment response, establish a prognosis, or to determine infection status. Performing an individual diagnostic test is technical; however, its interpretation and contextualization requires medical and epidemiologic skills that veterinary practitioners are able to master. This article shows the added value of the context of test prescription and correct interpretation highlighting the central role of the veterinary practitioner.

> Veterinarians may be asked to assess the presence, absence, or prevalence of a disease in an animal population or to compare the effects of management factors on disease status or production performance. The scope of diagnostic investigations in ruminant populations is often limited by the availability of time, money, and animal handling infrastructure. Selecting the correct number and type of animals to sample maximizes the benefits of the investigation, while minimizing costs. To meet the objectives of the study, the veterinarian must understand the statistical elements that need to be considered to calculate the appropriate sample size.

> The reliability of clinical pathology laboratory results is directly related to the sample quality submitted. As such, clinicians must submit the most representative and highest quality sample possible by acquiring, handling, preparing, and shipping samples with utmost care. Cytology and blood smear slides should be evaluated for sufficient densities of intact, well-spread, nucleated cells before submission. Poorly prepared samples may delay or negate results, incurring unnecessary costs for the client and practice. Additionally, all practices should have quality assurance programs that include monitoring of equipment to minimize reporting errors. Maximizing resources is the name of the game!.

Laboratory testing is one part of clinical diagnosis, and quick and reliable testing results provide important data to support treatment decision and develop control strategies. Clinical viral testing has been shifting from traditional virus isolation and electron microscopy to molecular polymerase chain reaction and point-of-care antigen tests. This shift in diagnostic methodology also means change from looking for infectious virions or viral particles to hunting viral antigens and genomes. With technological development, it is predicted that metagenomic sequencing will be commonly used in veterinary clinical diagnosis for unveiling the whole picture of microbes involved in diseases in the future.

Serologic diagnosis is used to identify evidence of infection or vaccination by specific agents, or for population surveillance. The enzyme-linked immunosorbent assay and the serum (virus) neutralizing tests are most used for bovine serologic diagnosis. Although infectious agent-specific antibodies may include immunoglobulin M, immunoglobulin G, and immunoglobulin A, the antibody class is rarely specifically identified in diagnostic laboratory testing. When interpreting the results of serology, consider whether the antibodies are due to an agent that causes lifelong infection, transient infection with no history of vaccination, or transient infection with a history of vaccination. Paired serology is necessary to confirm recent infection in cattle with a history of vaccination.

Knowing how to effectively use veterinary diagnostic toxicology laboratories is key when navigating suspect toxicoses in ruminants. This begins with establishing a causal relationship between clinical signs and potential sources of exposure, followed by collecting the appropriate samples for toxicology testing. There are times in which a successful diagnosis is hindered by not obtaining a thorough case history and not knowing what specimens to collect, or how much specimen to submit, for toxicology testing. This article is intended to offer some guidance with respect to the effective use of veterinary toxicology/analytical chemistry laboratories when navigating suspect toxicology cases in ruminants.

Next-generation sequencing (NGS) was initially developed to aid sequencing of the human genome. This molecular method is cost effective for sequencing and characterizing genomes, not only those of humans or animals but also those of bacteria and other pathogens. However, rather than sequencing a single organism, a targeted NGS method can be used to specifically amplify pathogens of interest in a clinical sample for detection and characterization by sequencing. Targeted NGS is an ideal method for ruminant syndromic testing due to its ability to detect a variety of pathogens in a sample with a single test.

John Dustin Loy, Jessie D. Monday, and David R. Smith

Diagnostic advances such as next-generation sequencing, highly multiplexed real-time PCR tests, and MALDI-TOF mass spectrometry have provided a tremendous increase in the amount of diagnostic information to clinicians. However, interpretation and application of these results to both individual and herd-level diagnostics still require the necessary skills in critical thinking and diagnostic interpretation to maximize benefit. This article provides a summary of advancements in diagnostic medicine and interpretation, as well as identifies gaps in knowledge that can be targeted to continue to build on best practices and application of diagnostic tools to improve ruminant health.

VETERINARY CLINICS OF NORTH AMERICA: FOOD ANIMAL PRACTICE

THE CLINICS ARE NOW AVAILABLE ONLINE!
Access your subscription at:
www.theclinics.com

Preface

Ruminant Diagnostics: Emerging and Classical Approaches to Individuals and Populations

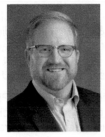
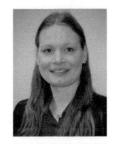
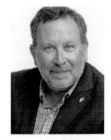

John Dustin Loy, DVM, PhD   Jessie D. Monday, DVM, MS   David R. Smith, DVM, PhD
Editors

Making a diagnosis is principal to medicine and precedes all other medical acts. Diagnostic testing is a critically important tool to help veterinarians diagnose disease or other medical conditions in clinical and population medicine. Livestock producers and veterinarians depend on accurate diagnostic information to explain clinical signs, rule at-risk diseases in or out, inform treatment and prevention strategies, provide a prognosis, and ultimately improve animal health and well-being. New methods and techniques, such as PCR, sequencing, and mass spectrometry, have revolutionized the amount and types of information that are available to clinicians on diagnostic reports. In the meantime, classical approaches, such as culture and serology, remain critical methods of disease investigation and risk management. The partnership between laboratorians, clinicians, and producers in utilizing diagnostics is becoming ever more important as a mix of new and classical diagnostic methodologies provides increased diagnostic sensitivity as well as result interpretation challenges.

In ruminant medicine, clinicians are tasked with not only making a diagnosis regarding the health condition of individual animals but also applying diagnostic findings to populations such as herds and flocks. This issue focuses on advances in diagnostic medicine and classical approaches to diagnostic medicine and has an emphasis on applying diagnostic findings to populations.

We truly appreciate all the authors, which include epidemiologists, internal medicine specialists, preventive medicine experts, microbiologists, immunologists, clinical and anatomical pathologists, pharmacologists, and toxicologists, among many others, for their contributions to this issue. We hope this issue provides an update and

Vet Clin Food Anim 39 (2023) xiii–xiv
https://doi.org/10.1016/j.cvfa.2022.12.001
0749-0720/23/© 2022 Published by Elsevier Inc.

reference on diagnostics to those working in ruminant medicine, and we are certain there is something for everyone within.

John Dustin Loy, DVM, PhD
Nebraska Veterinary Diagnostic Center
School of Veterinary Medicine and
Biomedical Sciences
University of Nebraska–Lincoln
4040 East Campus Loop N
Lincoln, NE 68583-0907, USA

Jessie D. Monday, DVM, MS
Texas A&M Veterinary Medical
Diagnostic Laboratory–Canyon
WT Box 60818
Canyon, TX 79016, USA

David R. Smith, DVM, PhD
College of Veterinary Medicine
Mississippi State University
240 Wise Center Drive
PO Box 6100
Mississippi State, MS 39762, USA

E-mail addresses:
jdloy@unl.edu (J.D. Loy)
jessie.Monday@tvmdl.tamu.edu (J.D. Monday)
david.smith@msstate.edu (D.R. Smith)

Interpretation and Analysis of Individual Diagnostic Tests and Performance

Sébastien Buczinski, Dr Vét, MSc[a],*, Simon Dufour, DMV, PhD[b],
Juan Carlos Arango-Sabogal, DMV, PhD[b]

KEYWORDS

- Clinical decision making • Bayes rule • Accuracy • Test prescription

KEY POINTS

- Sensitivity and specificity are key diagnostic test metrics that estimation needs to account for various types of biases and imperfect reference standard tests.
- Sensitive diagnostic tests help in ruling out disease when a negative test result is obtained (sensitive test/negative result/rule out).
- Specific diagnostic tests help in ruling in disease when a positive test result is obtained (specific test/positive result/rule in).
- Pretest probability of the disease helps to get an updated posttest probability of disease based on test results.
- Diagnostic test accuracy studies come with various challenges (biases, study design) that need to be appraised carefully to put in perspective the reported sensitivity and specificity.

Diagnostic tests are used daily in food animal veterinary practice. The word diagnostic originates from the Ancient Greek term "diagnôstikôs," which means "able to distinguish." In the current interpretation of diagnostic tests in veterinary medicine, we try to distinguish sick from nonsick animals, infected versus noninfected animals, or more generally the presence or absence of a given target condition. A test is defined as a tool or process aimed at detecting or quantifying a causal agent, clinical signs, lesions, or immune response in an individual, but also at determining the risk of being infected (eg, by using a risk assessment questionnaire).[1] Tests are used for screening or for diagnosis purposes depending on the stage of the disease in which they are applied. When tests are used to confirm a disease or guide a treatment, they are called

Disclosure: The authors have nothing to disclose.
[a] Département des Sciences Cliniques, Faculté de Médecine Vétérinaire, Université de Montréal, 3200 Rue Sicotte, St-Hyacinthe, Québec J2S 2M2, Canada; [b] Département de Pathologie et Microbiologie, Faculté de Médecine Vétérinaire, Université de Montréal, 3200 Rue Sicotte, St-Hyacinthe, Québec J2S 2M2, Canada
* Corresponding author.
E-mail address: s.buczinski@umontreal.ca

diagnostic tests.[1] Sometimes, tests are used to help determine the prognosis of a clinical process; thus, by extension, they are considered as specific cases of diagnostic tests where the objective is not to diagnose a medical condition, but to determine if a poor versus good outcome would occur. In this latter condition, the term "prognostic test" is more appropriate than diagnostic test, because the test is used to predict an event that is yet to happen (ie, a future outcome). Diagnostic tests are performed at the individual level for direct application on the sampled individual and for various purposes (**Box 1**).

However, when a test is used in an apparently healthy individual or population to systematically search for a condition (infection, immune reaction, or causative agent) that had previously gone unnoticed, it is called a screening test.[1] Screening tests can also be performed as part of strategies to meet a population objective and need to take into account such factors as the economic impact of the disease and the costs and performance (sensitivity and specificity) of the tests.[2] When applied to a population (vs an individual), they are interpreted at the herd level, either based on tests of multiple individual (eg, serology of multiple cows to determine the infection status of the herd), pooled individual samples (eg, milk bulk tank), or at the subgroup level (eg, sampling pen bedding). We restrict our discussion on individual samples and individual interpretation. For herd level tests, please refer to the Elizabeth Parker's article, "Diagnostic Strategies for Ruminant Populations," elsewhere in this issue.

TEST PERFORMANCE INTERPRETATION AND EXPLANATION

Starting with a simple example, a diagnostic test helps to distinguish two or more health statuses. For example, tests are used for detecting a given pathogen in a cow or the presence of clinical and paraclinical signs associated with disease. Starting from a basic clinical perspective, the percussion and auscultation of the right caudal thorax and abdomen of dairy cows is a test used to detect right displaced abomasum-abomasal volvulus (RDA-AV). The presence of a "ping" could be defined as a positive test result and the absence as a negative test result. Apart from the interoperator variation (**Box 2**), the presence of a ping would be used to confirm the RDA-AV diagnosis. However, not all cows with RDA-AV have a positive test (eg, no audible ping in cows with RDA-AV with a small liquid-gas interface or a thick abdominal wall).

The sensitivity of the test is defined as the proportion of animals with the target condition (here RDA-AV) that have a positive test result (ping). False-negative animals are animals with RDA-AV that have a negative test result (no ping). The specificity of a test is defined as the proportion of animals without the target condition that are classified as negative by the test (ie, cows without RDA-AV that have no ping). However, the presence of ping can also be found in cows without RDA-AV (eg, cows with various gastrointestinal disorders). The cows without RDA-AV with a positive test result are called false positive. These different concepts are illustrated in **Table 1** and can be extended for any diagnostic test and target condition. The definition of the target condition is generally a medical or surgical condition, but can be extended to any feature that is diagnosed (eg, detection of pregnancy or good quality colostrum). The ideal test would be a test that has high sensitivity (few false negative results) and high specificity (few false positive results). However, tests can also be of clinical interest when only one of the two parameters is high or even with moderate accuracy. For instance, a negative result from a highly sensitive test (>95%) is helpful to rule out a disease (sensitive test/negative result/rule out). In this case, the proportion of diseased animals with a negative result (false negative) is likely to be small given the high sensitivity of the test. Therefore, there is a high

Box 1
Specific examples and contexts when diagnostic tests can be used in cattle practice

Individual

- Individual animal and individual test

Why?	Example	Context of Test Use
Make a diagnosis	Isolation of bovine respiratory syncytial virus in a steer with bovine respiratory disease symptoms (herd not recently vaccinated with modified live virus).	Diagnosis
Confirm a suspicion	Early lactating, low-producing, anorectic cow (diagnostic test = auscultation and percussion of the left abdomen to confirm a left displaced abomasum diagnosis).	Diagnosis
Rule in or rule out a condition to select patient for a secondary test	A negative result to serum enzyme-linked immunosorbent assay in a cow with clinical signs of enzootic leukosis helps to rule out bovine leukosis virus implication.	Diagnosis
Monitoring treatment response or prognostic test	Serum creatine kinase measurement to determine the risk of nonrecovery in downer cows. Creatine kinase helps quantify the progression of muscle damage during treatment.	Prognosis/diagnosis
Determine infection status	Bovine viral diarrhea virus detection in a healthy-appearing calf before introduction in a herd.	Screening/diagnosis

- Strategies combining results of 2 independent tests

	Impact on the Accuracy of the Diagnostic Process		
Interpretation	Sensitivity	Specificity	Use
Parallel	Increases the sensitivity: sensitivity of the process *is at least equal or higher* than the sensitivity of the *most sensitive test*	Decreases the specificity: specificity of the process *is at most equal or lower* than the specificity of the *less specific test*	Rule out disease (sensitive test/negative result/rule out)

| Series | Decreases the sensitivity: sensitivity of the process is *at most equal or lower* than the sensitivity of the *less sensitive* test | Increases the specificity: specificity of the process *is at least equal or higher* than the specificity of the *most specific* test | Rule in the disease (specific test/positive result/rule in) |

- Using a second test based on a first test result in the same animal

Using a particular test depending on an initial test result can also be used in practice (sequential testing). For example, after performing a California Mastitis Test, we can then decide to perform a milk bacteriologic culture on those samples collected from quarters with increased somatic cell counts.

Herd or group-level tests

Why?	How	Example
Determination of a herd indicator based on individual tests	Performing individual tests in multiple individuals and interpretation based on the proportion of normal/abnormal tests	Quantifying the prevalence of adequate transfer of passive immunity in calves, of hyperketonemia in early lactating cows, or of subacute ruminal acidosis
Determination of herd infection status	Determining herd status by pooling samples from multiple animals	Bulk milk sample analysis for various infectious pathogens (eg, *Salmonella Dublin*, bovine leukosis virus, *Mycoplasma bovis*) Environmental sampling for *Mycobacterium avium* subsp. *paratuberculosis* detection
Establishing the prevalence of a specific disease or determining if a herd is free of a specific disease	Use of diagnostic tests to establish the within-herd prevalence or to rule out the presence of the disease in a herd	Multiple or all individuals are sampled for establishing the prevalence of the disease or infection or to determine the probability of disease freedom in a population (based on test accuracy and sample size calculation)

Box 2			
Agreement and reliability of diagnostic tests			
Type of Measurement	**Type of Test**	**Source of Errors**	**Reliability Indicators**
Continuous	Laboratory test, physical examination test (eg, heart rate, body temperature)	Patient or sample characteristics, device used for measurement, sampling technique and storage, operator performing the examination	Coefficient of variation, intraclass correlation coefficient
Categorical (dichotomous, polytomous, ordinal)	Imaging test, clinical score, milk bacteriology, physical examination test (eg, presence of a ping, presence of nasal discharge, body condition score)	Patient characteristics, device used for measurement, operator performing the examination	Percentage of agreement, Kappa and Kappa-like indicators, other indicators adjusted for the agreement beyond chance

Before using a diagnostic test in practice, it is important to know the sources of variation that are present beyond the specific patients' characteristics. For continuous measurements, it is also important to determine the impact of the rater/device variability versus the variability of the measurement. For categorical measurements, the agreement beyond chance (ie, different from raw percentage of agreement) is generally required to know if the score or measurement is robust to rater classification. It is also important to notice that none of the reliability indicators is perfect and that we should not rely on only one of these indicators.

probability that the negative test result obtained from a highly sensitive test originates from a nondiseased animal (ie, a high negative predictive value [NPV]; discussed in a subsequent section). A positive result from a highly specific test is useful to rule in a disease (specific test/positive result/rule in) given that the probability of observing false-positive results from highly specific test is likely low. Tests with moderate accuracy may also be helpful in the clinical decision-making process. However, in these situations, it is crucial to also have in mind the clinical context of test application together with a good understanding of the patient's clinical characteristics.

Sometimes, a diagnostic strategy involving multiples tests is used to increase the accuracy of the entire diagnostic process (see **Box 1**). For instance, the test results of two tests performed on the same individual can be combined and interpreted in parallel or in series. In parallel interpretation, the individual would be considered positive if a positive result to either test is observed. This approach is used when the consequences of false-negative results (ie, missing a diseased individual) are more important than false-positive results. Because parallel interpretation increases the sensitivity of the diagnostic process, it is used when we want to rule out the disease (sensitive test/negative result/rule out). In series interpretation, the individual would be considered positive if a positive result to both tests is observed. This approach is used when the consequences of false-positive results (ie, misclassifying a healthy individual as positive) are more important than false-negative results. Because serial interpretation increases the specificity of the diagnostic process, it is used when we want to rule in the diseased (specific test/positive result/rule in). The impact of serial and parallel interpretation on the sensitivity and specificity of the diagnostic process is summarized in **Box 1**. For

Table 1
Intrinsic diagnostic test characteristics and accuracy metrics used in practice

Test results	Target Condition		
	Diseased	**Nondiseased**	
Positive test	TP	FP	
Negative test	FN	TN	
	$D = p*n$	$\bar{D} = (1-p)*n$	n

Intrinsic individual test metrics:

Sensitivity (Se): ability of the test to detect diseased animals. The sensitivity represents the proportion of animals with the target condition that tested positive, or the probability of a positive test result given that the disease is present.

$$Se = \frac{TP}{TP+FN}$$

Specificity (Sp): ability of the test to detect nondiseased animals. The specificity represents the proportion of animals without the target condition that tested negative, or the probability of a negative test result given that the disease is absent.

$$Sp = \frac{TN}{TN+FP}$$

Population-based metrics:

PLR is the proportion of diseased animals with a positive test versus proportion of nondiseased animals with a positive test.

$$PLR = \frac{P(T^+|D^+)}{P(T^+|D^-)} = \frac{Se}{(1-Sp)}$$

NLR is the proportion of diseased animals with a negative test versus proportion of nondiseased animals with a negative test.

$$NLR = \frac{P(T^-|D^+)}{P(T^-|D^-)} = \frac{(1-Se)}{Sp}$$

PPV is the probability that a positive test comes from a diseased animal in a specific population. Clinically it is interpreted as: how confident we can be that an animal that tested positive is a true positive.

$$PPV = \frac{TP}{TP+FP} = \frac{p*Se}{[p*Se+(1-p)*(1-Sp)]}$$

NPV is the probability that a negative test comes from a nondiseased animal in a specific population. Clinically it is interpreted as: how confident we can be that an animal that tested negative is a true negative.

$$NPV = \frac{TN}{TN+FN} = \frac{(1-p)*Sp}{[(1-p)*Sp+p*(1-Se)]}$$

As the sensitivity and specificity, PLR, and NLR are intrinsic characteristics of the tests, the predictive values provide information on its interpretation in a given population.

Abbreviations: D, number of animals with the target condition; $\bar{D}$, number of animals without the target condition; FN, false negative; FP, false positive; n, total sampled population; p, prevalence of the disease in the population; TN, true negative; TP, true positive.

independent tests, simple formulas are used to calculate the sensitivity and specificity of test results interpreted either in series or in parallel. Two tests A and B are considered independent when the probability of obtaining a given result to test A, for example, does not depend on the results from test B.[1]

Parallel interpretation: the individual is considered positive if a positive result to either test is observed.

$$Se_{parallel} = Se_{test\ A} + Se_{test\ B} - (Se_{test\ A} \times Se_{test\ B})$$

$$Sp_{parallel} = Sp_{test\ A} \times Sp_{test\ B}$$

Series interpretation: the individual is considered positive if a positive result to both tests is observed.

$$Se_{series} = Se_{test\ A} \times Se_{test\ B}$$

$$Sp_{series} = Sp_{test\ A} + Sp_{test\ B} - (Sp_{test\ A} \times Sp_{test\ B})$$

For nonindependent tests, a modification to the previous equations (eg, including a correlation between the tests) is required to calculate the sensitivity and specificity of serial and parallel interpretations. However, this calculation is beyond of the scope of this article.

ADEQUATE PRESCRIPTION OF THE TEST FOR AN ADEQUATE INTERPRETATION OF ITS RESULT

The example of the ping auscultation for RDA-AV detection is a simple clinical example. One can easily understand that the test result is influenced by the degree and nature of the abomasal content, therefore affecting the sensitivity of the test, or other abdominal organs, which may be associated with a ping sound in the absence of RDA-AV (eg, gas within intestinal lumen). The test accuracy may also be affected by other conditions, such as the cow body condition score with decreased possibility to find a ping in fat cows especially if the gas/liquid interface is small. Some conditions not related to the patient can also affect test accuracy. For example, in a noisy environment (close to a barn fan) the ability of the veterinarian to detect a ping can also be affected. Beyond these considerations, other conditions that are related to test reliability could also influence test accuracy (eg, the type of stethoscope used, veterinarian's ability for auscultation [see **Box 2**]). Therefore, the context where the diagnostic test is applied is paramount. Illustration of the importance of the context of test prescription is more easily judged in the case of a complex infectious disease, such as paratuberculosis, where laboratory tests can be prescribed and interpreted. **Fig. 1**A illustrates how fecal shedding, cell-mediated immune response, humoral response, and clinical signs typically progress over time in *Mycobacterium avium* subsp. *paratuberculosis*–infected cows. Based on this figure, we can imagine that a negative enzyme-linked immunosorbent assay (ELISA) test would not have the same meaning in a cow that could be on its early stage of infection, when humoral immunity is not developed, compared with a negative ELISA test in a cow with clinical signs of the disease (ie, emaciation and diarrhea with no significant impairment of the general status). In the case of this infectious disease, proper knowledge of the

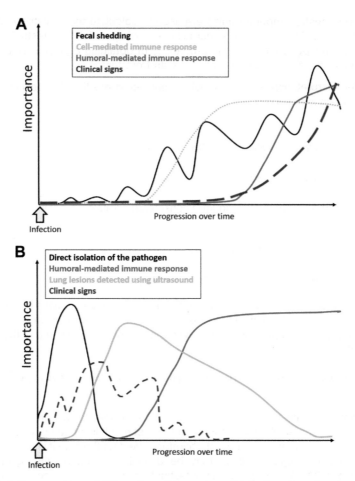

Fig. 1. Variation over time of different possible markers of infection status in cows suffering from (A) chronic infectious disease (eg, infected by *Mycobacterium avium* subsp. *paratuberculosis*) or (B) acute infectious disease (eg, infected by a bacteria involved in bronchopneumonia). One can note that some pathogens involved in bronchopneumonia are found before the onset of the disease because of healthy carriers in the upper respiratory tract. These figures are generic and the spikes of the curves are for illustrative purposes only.

pathophysiology of infection (as illustrated in **Fig. 1**A) would help the clinician to know which test has the highest chances of detecting the target condition depending on the clinical situation. In acute diseases (ie, acute viral or bacterial infection associated with bronchopneumonia) the dynamics of the different ancillary tests' positivity are different (**Fig. 1**B). In this context, the aspect of the test results dynamics over time may also change depending on the type of agent involved because some bacteria/agents are found in healthy carriers and antibodies or presence of viruses from recent modified live viruses vaccination may exist before infection depending on the vaccination and exposure status of the animal. These two simple examples illustrate the importance of the context of test prescription for a better interpretation of their results, which need a good knowledge of the pathophysiology of the target condition to diagnose.

USE OF DIAGNOSTIC TESTS IN CLINICAL REASONING: TEST AND TREATMENT THRESHOLDS

The use of diagnostic tests is generally associated with the need of making a decision and reducing the uncertainty associated with this decision. This theoretic strategy is illustrated in **Fig. 2**. Briefly, before performing any supplementary test, each target condition (eg, disease) that needs to be identified has a probability of being present in a patient. This probability is considered as the "best-guess" that the patient has the target condition based on the clinical presentation and context. For instance, after a proper examination process the veterinarian can determine that the probability is too low for warranting further investigation (eg, probability of limb fracture in a calf without lameness). Below this "test threshold," no test or action is required. However, if the clinical signs are obvious, the clinical diagnosis is evident, and no additional test is required to reach the final diagnosis (eg, probability of limb fracture in a lame calf with deformation and open fracture). Other tests, such as radiographs, can be performed for choosing the best treatment options (depending on the type and complexity of the bone fracture) but not for the diagnosis of the fracture per se. The treatment threshold defines the conditions where a diagnostic test is not required

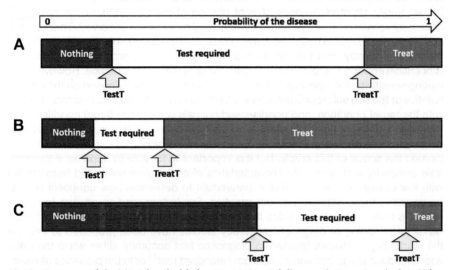

Fig. 2. Concepts of decision thresholds for treatment and diagnostic test prescription. When facing an animal with a possible suspicion of a disease, it is important to consider that the whole spectrum of the disease can be observed. For animals with a low probability of being affected by the disease, below this threshold, no further diagnostic test is required (test threshold [TestT]). Above the clinical suspicion (treatment threshold [TreatT]), no further test is required for establishing the diagnosis and a treatment is prescribed. The general framework (A) is adapted for any disease condition. In some circumstances, the TreatT is decreased if the target condition is common or if the treatment has limited consequences and can also provide information that can help with the diagnosis confirmation (B). For instance, a herd where left displaced abomasum is common and where a cow has all clinical signs of left displaced abomasum but the ping is observed. In this case, the explorative laparotomy for performing abomasopexy/omentopexy could potentially be prescribed without any supplementary tests. The TestT can also be raised (C) with high pretest probability of disease especially when the test is invasive or difficult to perform. For example, an echocardiography would not be performed in any cow with tachycardia in the absence of any other cardiac suspicion in physical examination or history.

because of the certainty of the diagnosis. The treatment threshold can also be influenced by the nature of the treatment required and its relative cost compared with the cost associated with the diagnostic test. These two thresholds depend on the disease to be diagnosed and the clinical context. Below the test threshold and above the treatment threshold, no diagnostic test is required. Ancillary tests can still be performed for characterizing the prognosis or targeting the best treatment option. Between these two thresholds, uncertainty is present and diagnostic tests are required to help the clinician in ruling in or ruling out a given disease.

KEY METRICS OF TEST ACCURACY: SENSITIVITY, SPECIFICITY, AND LIKELIHOOD RATIOS

Diagnostic tests are part of our daily clinical work-up as bovine practitioners. However, not all the diagnostic tests used in practice have published accuracy metrics relative to a given condition. For example, severe tachycardia is a predictor of prognosis in cows with RDA-AV.[3] However, the ability of the presence of severe tachycardia to diagnose cows with RDA-AV is not known and should be poor because of the lack of specificity of this clinical sign. For instance, cows with various conditions associated with pain, dehydration, or fever are tachycardic. On the opposite, the sensitivity would be negatively affected in cases of right dilation of the abomasum or in cows with abomasal volvulus in its early stage where normal heart rate is observed. The test metrics are generally driven by the sensitivity and specificity (see **Table 1**), which are by far the most frequently reported intrinsic test characteristics. Determination of their value is of critical importance to assess the usefulness of the test in practice. However, estimating sensitivity and specificity is not that easy because they depend on the characteristics of the two subpopulations on which the tests are applied (ie, diseased animals with the target condition, and nondiseased animals without the target condition). For this reason, different types of potential biases have been reported in studies assessing diagnostic test accuracy (**Table 2**). Extensive discussion of these types of bias is beyond the scope of this article, but it is important to be able to appraise if the available sensitivity and specificity characteristics of a test were estimated from studies with low or high risk of bias. This is paramount to determine how confident we can be on using these estimates in our practice. For further reading on that topic, the reader is referred to other articles from the medical[4–6] or veterinary fields.[7–10] Standards for reporting of diagnostic accuracy studies have been proposed to improve the readability of studies focused in diagnostic test accuracy either when the reference standard test is considered as a gold standard test[11] or in the presence of imperfect reference standard test.[12] These checklists are helpful for judging the strengths and weaknesses associated with these studies.

KEY METRICS OF TEST VALUE, WHEN APPLIED IN A GIVEN POPULATION

The positive predictive value (PPV) and NPV are two additional important test metrics (see **Table 2**). The predictive values are not intrinsic characteristics of the test itself, but rather characteristics of the test in the population where it is applied. This example is generally well illustrated by a test for detecting infectious agents in a specific population where some information on the prevalence of the infection is known. Predictive values represent the probability that a positive (or negative) test came from a truly positive (or truly negative) animal. Consider the two scenarios presented in **Fig. 3**. In scenario A, a test with a sensitivity of 90% and a specificity of 95% was applied to a population where 5% of the animals were truly diseased. In scenario B, the exact same test was applied in a population where prevalence of disease was 30%, thus

Table 2
Potential bias associated with the determination of diagnostic test accuracy (sensitivity and specificity) depending on the index test and the reference standard test characteristics

Type of Bias	Implication for the Accuracy of the Test of Interest	Solution to Limit This Risk of Bias
Classification bias/ imperfect reference standard	If the index test (test of interest) is compared with an imperfect reference standard, sensitivity and specificity estimates could be biased because any discrepancy between the index test and reference standard is, by default, considered as an error of the index test.	Considering the absence of gold standard/reference standard in the accuracy estimation method (using latent class models), using panel-based classification with panelists reviewing all patients' characteristics to increase the confidence in the classification or changing the reference standard to a gold standard test when possible.
Spectrum of the disease/selection bias	Animals with the target condition are classified by a specific finding and animals without the target condition are classified with another case definition that is not mutually exclusive from the first one. This allows for the selection of patients at the extremity of the disease spectrum (see **Fig. 2**A). This selection artificially inflates the accuracy estimates excluding cases in the midspectrum of the disease	Only one mutually exclusive definition of the target disease condition should be allowed. This defines the "one-gate" study design where all the samples of interest are submitted to the same test (positive or negative).
Verification bias (work-up or referral bias)	Comes from studies where patients are selected for the reference standard test only if they have undergone the index test. This selection leads to a lack of generalizability of the study (ie, only more severe cases could be submitted to the index test then biasing the findings toward this higher risk population).	The study design should be determined a priori in an adequate manner to limit this impact.
Incorporation bias	Comes from studies where the index test is part of the reference standard definition. An example is to determine the optimal size of cavitary mass to detect lung abscesses looking on a database where the diagnosis was based on radiograph reading. The aspect of lung radiograph is the reference standard that includes part of the index test results.	Sometimes difficult to avoid based on the difference between the index test and the reference standard. If possible, changing the reference standard could be useful.
Observer or test review bias	If the observer performing the index test knows the reference standard test result, it could bias (even if not intentionally) the	Adequate blinding should be used when possible. For example, interpretation of thoracic ultrasound cannot be performed

(continued on next page)

Table 2 (continued)		
Type of Bias	Implication for the Accuracy of the Test of Interest	Solution to Limit This Risk of Bias
	findings toward better accuracy of the index test. This would not be possible, although for a very objective index test (eg, measurement of a blood metabolite).	without looking to the patient (eg, calf with severe dyspnea and clinical signs of bovine respiratory disease). In this case, the observer can interpret the same image differently versus an examination performed in a calf with no obvious clinical signs.
Differential reference bias	Comes from studies where different reference standard tests are applied to the sample of patients. For example, a new biomarker to detect endocarditis in cows could be tested in a population of cows where some cows are confirmed with endocarditis using necropsy, whereas others are confirmed using echocardiography.	The accuracy observed may depend on the difference between the two reference standard tests used. Again here, the latent class model approach, which compares all tests as if they were imperfect, could help solve this issue.
Important delay between index test and reference standard (temporal bias)	If the delay between the index test and the reference standard test is important, misclassification may occur because of the natural progression of the target condition (eg, necropsy to confirm a target condition a few wk/mo after performing a blood sample analysis for a specific biomarker, or serum ELISA and individual fecal culture test performed at different times for paratuberculosis diagnosis in a cow).	The maximal acceptable interval between the index test and the reference standard test should be defined a priori during the study design. Alternatively, probability of cure or of having an incident event between tests can be incorporated in a latent class model analytical strategy.

a considerably higher prevalence. For the low prevalence scenario (see **Fig. 3**A), we can see that most test-positive animals were actually false-positive results. Indeed, within the animals that tested positive, we actually have more false-positive (n = 11), than true-positive (n = 6). In that example, the actual PPV was 35% (6/17), which is interpreted as: in this population, there is a 35% chance that a test-positive animal is truly diseased. However, we could be certain that test-negative animals were truly negative. Indeed, we had only eight false-negative among the 183 individuals that tested negative (thus an NPV of 96%). Note that the theoretic PPV and NPV, based on the formula proposed in **Table 2**, would be 49% and 99%, respectively (in this example, we applied a stochastic process where each true positive animal had 90% chance of testing positive, and each truly healthy animal had 95% chance of testing negative; thus we did not get exactly 90% and 95% of animals being distributed in each group). Despite that the exact same test was applied in the high-prevalence population (see **Fig. 3**B), the proportions of truly healthy versus diseased individuals in the test-positive and test-negative individuals are strikingly different. Within the test-positive animals, we now have 62 out of 67 (93%) that were truly

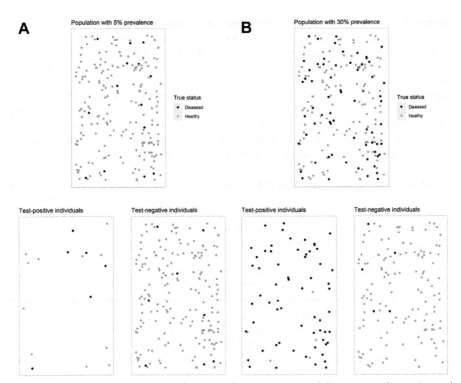

Fig. 3. Illustration of test results as function of test accuracy and disease prevalence. Beyond the test accuracy, the prevalence of disease in a population is also an important determinant of the predictive value of a test. This figure illustrates the probability that a positive (or negative) test came from a truly positive (or truly negative) animal. In scenario A, a test with a sensitivity of 90% and a specificity of 95% was applied to a population where 5% of the animals were truly diseased (*top box*). We can easily see that most of the test-positive animals (*bottom left box*) were false-positive indicating a low PPV for that test, in this population. In scenario B, the exact same test was applied in a population where prevalence of disease was 30% (*top box*). In that latter population, the test had excellent PPV and NPV (ie, in that population, we can be certain of the status of an animal, based on its test result).

diseased. Among test-negative animals, 128 out of 133 (95%) were correctly classified (and the theoretic PPV and NPV would be 89% and 96%, respectively). So, the exact same test performed better, in term of its predictive abilities, when applied to the population with the higher disease prevalence. The fact that predictive values of a test vary as function of the population within which it is applied is important to grasp for correct interpretation of a diagnostic test result. We dive further into this in the following section.

HOW TO INCORPORATE TEST ACCURACY TO DETERMINE THE FINAL DIAGNOSIS AFTER KNOWING THE TEST RESULTS IN AN INDIVIDUAL: USING CLINICAL REASONING (BAYES RULE)

Knowing the context in which the prescription is made is not the only important thing to decide which test to propose for a given condition. The clinician should also have a prior idea of the probability that the animal has the target condition or disease before performing a test. This concept, also known as pretest probability of the disease, is intuitively used in practice but generally not properly expressed as such. This probability is expressed as the estimated proportion of patients with the same clinical characteristics that really have the target condition. The reader can note here that the patients we are referring here for defining pretest probability are the hypothetical patients with the same presentation and clinical signs (which is different from the population approach used for illustrating PPV and NPV). This approach is inherent to the use of likelihood ratios (LR) of the test or Bayes rule application, which update pretest probability based on the test result into a posttest probability.[13,14] The difference between the pretest and posttest probability is literally interpreted as the added value of the diagnostic test in the clinical work-up.

Coming back to the example of the cow tested for paratuberculosis, the impact of a negative result in a cow with a very low suspicion of the disease based on clinical examination is not the same than in a cow with all the clinical characteristics findings. In **Table 1**, test metrics called LR of a test result (either positive LR [PLR] or negative LR [NLR]) are defined. These ratios only depend on test specificity and sensitivity and are therefore free of prevalence context by contrast to predictive values (see **Table 1**). These ratios indicate how likelier it is to observe a given test result (positive for PLR or negative for NLR) in diseased versus nondiseased animals. The higher the PLR the better the test is to rule in the disease in the presence of a positive test. The lower the NLR the better the test is for ruling out a disease in the presence of a negative test result. As a rule of thumb, clinically relevant tests should generally have a PLR greater than 10, and NLR less than 0.1.[15] The Bayes theorem links the pretest probability ($P_{pretest}$) to the posttest probability ($P_{posttest}$) of the disease through the following formula:

Posttest odds = Pretest odds * Likelihood ratio;

where odds = p/(1-p) and after a little math gives a slightly more complicated formula linking posttest probability to pretest probability and LR:

$$P_{post-test} = \frac{P_{pretest}}{LR/\left(\left[1 - P_{pretest}\right] + \left[P_{pretest} * LR\right]\right)}$$

In our example of the cow with suspicion of clinical paratuberculosis, if the practitioner wants to diagnose the disease based on a simple blood sample, we can consider that ELISA test on blood has a low sensitivity and high specificity with most probable estimates being 27% and 97%, respectively, as reported in a previous study.[16] The added value of the test in the diagnostic pathway heavily depends on the pretest probability that the animal has the disease as illustrated in **Fig. 4** using a Fagan nomogram. This visual representation combines the pretest probability (illustrated as the point on the left y-axis from which both lines are emanating) and LR of the test (reported as PLR and NLR on the top right corner of the figure) to determine the posttest probability for a test-negative (illustrated as the end of the blue line on the right y-axis) or test-positive animal (illustrated as the end of the red line on the right y-axis[17,18]). The pretest probability is closely related to the concept of the expected prevalence of the target condition in individual animals with the same clinical characteristics. The pretest probability is defined as the expected percentage of animals presenting the same clinical profile that would be truly infected (ie, with the target condition to diagnose). This information rarely exists in practice. However, it can be approximated based on the clinician's clinical experience or previous studies conducted in the same type of animals. Here is where the knowledge of the disease presentation and the differential diagnoses, in combination with clinical assessment of the animal are important. For example, if a cow has a low probability of being affected by paratuberculosis based on the absence of obvious clinical signs, the expected pretest probability could be anticipated as no higher than the expected prevalence of the disease in the average population of cows. In the province of Québec, this prevalence would be at the cow level lower than 5%,[16] thus, the conservative scenario of 5% used for illustration in **Fig. 4** scenario A. This scenario would also depend on the herd history. For instance, one might expect a higher pretest probability in herds with history of clinical cases of paratuberculosis compared with herds with no history of the disease. Then, one could imagine the situation where there are roughly equal chances (50%) of having the disease (see **Fig. 4** scenario B). Finally, the test could also be performed in a cow with a high pretest probability of the disease (eg, a thin cow with chronic diarrhea, no fever, normal appetite, no history of gastrointestinal parasitism, and housed in a herd where the disease was previously diagnosed). In this situation, we could imagine a higher pretest probability (75%) as illustrated in **Fig. 4** scenario C. These situations represent three different scenarios with low, mid, and high pretest probability of the disease using the same test (serum ELISA test). A nomogram is used to visualize the incremental value of the test based on the pretest probability and the PLR or NLR. The added value of the test is seen as the difference between the pretest and posttest probability. This change of probability (between pretest and posttest) is seen as the new information given by the test result. For a specific test, such as the ELISA for paratuberculosis, we can see that a positive test is rapidly increasing the posttest probability of the disease because of the low false-positive rate of the disease. However, this increase depends on the pretest probability. In a low pretest probability setting (see **Fig. 4** scenario A), this increase is moderate, with a rise from 5% to 32% chances of truly having paratuberculosis. However, with a high pretest probability of disease (see **Fig. 4** scenario C), a negative result does not affect much the probability of disease. A cow with 75% pretest probability of the disease would still have 69% probability of being affected after a negative ELISA test is performed (because ELISA has a low sensitivity). This example puts in perspective the test interpretation based on the condition of prescription of the test. With the same results (either positive or negative), the clinician would do different things based on the type of pretest probability associated with the context where the test is applied.

In various clinical conditions, the accuracy of the tests we use are far from having either a perfect sensitivity or specificity. The Wisconsin clinical scoring system was developed for helping to diagnose lower respiratory tract infection in dairy calves[19] and its accuracy has been previously estimated.[20] When using a score of 5 or more as a positive result, the sensitivity was 62.4% (95% bayesian credible intervals: 47.9–75.8) and specificity 74.1% (95% bayesian credible intervals: 64.9–82.8). The impact of a positive or negative test is seen in **Fig. 5** using, again, pretest probabilities of 5%, 50%, and 75%. Because of the low accuracy of the clinical test used, we can easily see that the added value of the test is limited and that, in most scenarios, this score should be complemented with another test to reach an adequate decision at the individual level. Luckily, applying a test, such as the Wisconsin clinical scoring system, is inexpensive. This explains why it is commonly applied, despite its moderate accuracy.

Using different "what if" scenarios for various possible pretest probabilities may also be helpful, especially because the exact determination of the true pretest probability may be challenging depending on the clinical context and the clinician as previously seen in human medical field.[21,22]

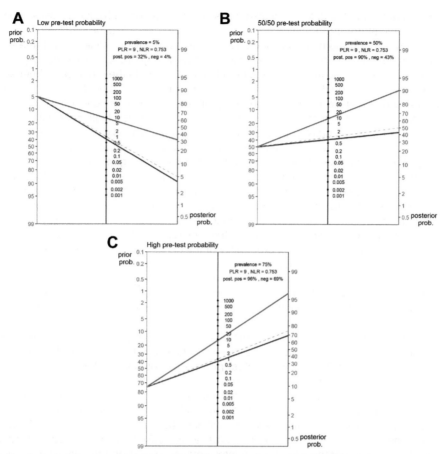

Fig. 4. Pretest and posttest probability of disease in a cow with paratuberculosis infection using ELISA test results and Bayes rule. Illustration of the relationship between pretest and posttest probabilities for three different scenarios with either a low (5%; *A*), medium (50%; *B*), or high (75%; *C*) pretest probability, and using the same test, an ELISA with sensitivity of 27% and specificity of 97%. The impact of test accuracy and pretest probability on posttest probability is represented in blue for a negative test and in red for a positive test. The dotted line delineates the pretest probability.

HOW TO USE BAYES RULE IN PRACTICE: USING CELL PHONE FREE APPS AND TESTS WITH KNOWN ACCURACY PARAMETERS

To use the Bayes rule, we need some information on test LR (or test sensitivity and specificity) and to determine the most plausible pretest probability. The hand calculation of the updated probability of disease after performing the test is a challenge because the equation is not easy to solve rapidly. However, the posttest probability is easily obtained from cell phone applications or online calculators.[13] For instance, World Wide Web interfaces (http://araw.mede.uic.edu/cgi-bin/testcalc.pl) and mobile applications (DocNomo; https://apps.apple.com/us/app/docnomo/id901279945; only available for the iOs platform) were developed to help practitioners compute posttest probabilities on the spot. These applications help the clinician to compute a quantitative assessment of the probability update either before choosing a test (ie, to evaluate what would be the gain from using this test) or after obtaining the

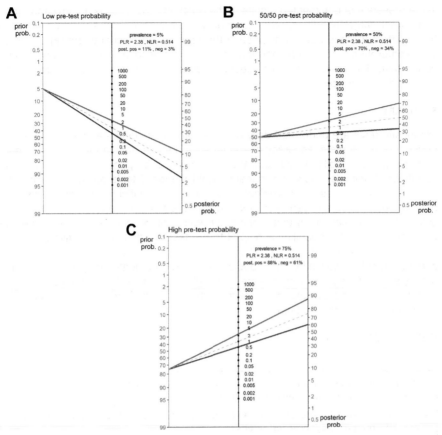

Fig. 5. Pretest and posttest probability of disease in a calf with bronchopneumonia using Wisconsin clinical respiratory score test results and Bayes rule. Illustration of the relationship between pretest and posttest probabilities for three different scenarios with either a low (5%; *A*), medium (50%; *B*), or high (75%; *C*) pretest probability, and using a same test, the Wisconsin clinical respiratory score (sensitivity, 62%; specificity, 74%). The impact of test accuracy and pretest probability on posttest probability is represented in blue for a negative test and in red for a positive test. The dotted line delineates the pretest probability.

test result (ie, for quantifying how previous knowledge should be updated by the obtained result). This reinforces the importance of a good knowledge of the context where the test would be applied and more specifically the physical examination of the patient. This examination process helps to "guess" the expected pretest probability that the patient has the target condition. Then, the diagnostic test prescription is targeted based on the pretest characteristics. The knowledge of the accuracy of the diagnostic test to be used serves to update the pretest probability in the posttest probability of disease.

Moreover, the treatment threshold varies from one disease to another and depends on various conditions, such as the cost of misclassification of a false-positive or false-negative case (see **Fig. 2**). The nomogram may serve as an additional tool to help clinicians and producers to make decisions. This approach also helps to determine whether to continue with the diagnostic process despite a negative test result. In these situations, explaining Bayes rule may help to convince the farmer to investigate further in the presence of unexpected results. If the posttest probability is not low enough to rule out the target condition, other strategies or diagnostic tests should be used. All these different steps put in perspective the importance of characterizing accuracy of the different clinical and paraclinical tests that are used in practice, not only diagnostic tests for the diagnosis of infectious diseases but tests that are commonly used in daily practice.

SUMMARY

Diagnostic tests are performed daily by veterinary practitioners and for various purposes. For many tests, accuracy characteristics are available in the form of an estimated sensitivity (ability to detect affected animals) and specificity (ability to detect nonaffected animals). However, because gold standard tests are not available for many clinical diseases, the imperfect sensitivity and specificity can lead to misdiagnosis especially in the absence of a clear diagnostic test prescription context. Clearly establishing the reasons of test prescription based on a prior knowledge of the test probability (pretest probability) is helpful to put test results in perspective (eg, using Bayes rule). This clinical approach also emphasizes the validation of diagnostic test accuracy results. Making informed decisions based on validated diagnostic tests ultimately serves to improve patient care and well-being and to tailor antimicrobial use, and would also improve the image of the veterinary practitioner as an added-value for diagnostic test interpretation.

CLINICS CARE POINTS

- When interpreting a diagnostic test result, the context of prescription (pretest probability of disease at the individual level) needs to be considered.
- A complete physical examination and an analysis of the population context is paramount to correctly interpret diagnostic test results.
- Depending on the prescription context, highly sensitive (rule in a disease) or highly specific tests (rule out a disease) could be used.

REFERENCES

1. Dohoo IR, Martin W, Stryhn HE. Veterinary epidemiologic research. Charlottetown: VER Inc; 2009.
2. Rothman KJ, Greenland S, Lash TL. Modern epidemiology. Wolters Kluwer health. Philadelphia: Lippincott Williams & Wilkins; 2008.
3. Boulay G, Francoz D, Dore E, et al. Preoperative cow-side lactatemia measurement predicts negative outcome in Holstein dairy cattle with right abomasal disorders. J Dairy Sci 2014;97:212–21.
4. Schmidt RL, Factor RE. Understanding sources of bias in diagnostic accuracy studies. Arch Pathol Lab Med 2013;137:558–65.
5. Schiller I, van Smeden M, Hadgu A, et al. Bias due to composite reference standards in diagnostic accuracy studies. Stat Med 2016;35:1454–70.
6. Willis BH. Spectrum bias: why clinicians need to be cautious when applying diagnostic test studies. Fam Pract 2008;25:390–6.
7. Buczinski S, O'Connor AM. Specific challenges in conducting and reporting studies on the diagnostic accuracy of ultrasonography in bovine medicine. Vet Clin North Am Food Anim Pract 2016;32:1–18.

8. Cheung A, Dufour S, Jones G, et al. Bayesian latent class analysis when the reference test is imperfect. Rev Sci Tech 2021;40:271–86.

9. Buczinski S, Pardon B. Bovine respiratory disease diagnosis: what progress has been made in clinical diagnosis? Vet Clin North Am Food Anim Pract 2020;36: 399–423.

10. Greiner M, Gardner IA. Epidemiologic issues in the validation of veterinary diagnostic tests. Prev Vet Med 2000;45:3–22.

11. Bossuyt PM, Reitsma JB, Bruns DE, et al. STARD 2015: an updated list of essential items for reporting diagnostic accuracy studies. Radiology 2015;277:826–32.

12. Kostoulas P, Nielsen SS, Branscum AJ, et al. STARD-BLCM: standards for the reporting of diagnostic accuracy studies that use bayesian latent class models. Prev Vet Med 2017;138:37–47.

13. Timsit E, Leguillette R, White BJ, et al. Likelihood ratios: an intuitive tool for incorporating diagnostic test results into decision-making. J Am Vet Med Assoc 2018; 252:1362–6.

14. Gardner IA. The utility of Bayes' theorem and bayesian inference in veterinary clinical practice and research. Aus Vet J 2002;80:758–61.

15. Grimes DA, Schulz KF. Refining clinical diagnosis with likelihood ratios. Lancet 2005;365:1500–5.

16. Arango-Sabogal JC, Fecteau G, Paré J, et al. Estimating diagnostic accuracy of fecal culture in liquid media for the detection of *Mycobacterium avium* subsp. *paratuberculosis* infections in Québec dairy cows: a latent class model. Prev Vet Med 2018;160:26–34.

17. Caraguel CG, Vanderstichel R. The two-step Fagan's nomogram: ad hoc interpretation of a diagnostic test result without calculation. Evid Based Med 2013;18: 125–8.

18. Fagan TJ. Letter: nomogram for Bayes theorem. New Engl J Med 1975;293:257.

19. McGuirk SM. Disease management of dairy calves and heifers. Vet Clin North Am Food Anim Pract 2008;24:139–53.

20. Buczinski S, Ollivett TL, Dendukuri N. Bayesian estimation of the accuracy of the calf respiratory scoring chart and ultrasonography for the diagnosis of bovine respiratory disease in pre-weaned dairy calves. Prev Vet Med 2015;119:227–31.

21. Phelps MA, Levitt MA. Pretest probability estimates: a pitfall to the clinical utility of evidence-based medicine? Acad Emerg Med 2004;11:692–4.

22. Bianchi MT, Alexander BM, Cash SS. Incorporating uncertainty into medical decision making: an approach to unexpected test results. Med Dec Mak 2009;29: 116–24.

Diagnostic Strategies for Ruminant Populations

Elizabeth Parker, BVSc, MPH, PhD, DACVPM*

KEYWORDS

- Sample size • Cluster sampling • Sampling unit • Sampling frame • Variance
- Precision • Confidence

KEY POINTS

- Statistical and nonstatistical factors need to be considered when deciding on the best strategy to meet the objectives of a diagnostic investigation in a population of animals.
- The natural variability in the population and the required levels of confidence, precision, and power of the statistical test determine the sample size required.
- The availability of the time and money required to conduct the investigation, and of the resources required to uniquely identify, handle, and restrain the animals for examination and sample collection, often are the most important drivers of the disease investigation strategy.

INTRODUCTION

Veterinarians conduct clinical examinations on individual animals every day, sometimes taking samples for laboratory testing, to make decisions on the cause and treatment of adverse results. At the same time, they may be scanning the rest of the herd, checking body condition, and looking for lameness, respiratory disease, or diarrhea while also checking the environment, airflow, temperature, and feed and pasture quality. Any information gathering activity, clinical examinations, taking measurements, or collecting samples is considered a diagnostic test. Sometimes this information is collected from the entire population, a census. In large populations, however, a census is often not possible and collecting measurements from a subset or sample of the population is more convenient and practical. Before embarking on any diagnostic investigation in a ruminant population, the veterinarian and the producer must first agree on the diagnostic question, and how the results of the investigation will be used. The farmer and the veterinarian must also consider the availability of resources, including appropriate animal handling and restraint facilities, unique identification of all the animals or sampling units in the population of interest, and the time and money required for sampling and diagnostic tests.

Department of Veterinary Preventive Medicine, The Ohio State University, 1920 Coffey Road, Columbus, OH 43210, USA
* Corresponding author.
E-mail address: parker.1224@osu.edu

Vet Clin Food Anim 39 (2023) 21–31
https://doi.org/10.1016/j.cvfa.2022.10.002
0749-0720/23/© 2022 Elsevier Inc. All rights reserved.

vetfood.theclinics.com

Diagnostic test sensitivity (Se) and specificity (Sp) should also be considered when calculating the sample size. Generally, if all other diagnostic objectives remain the same, as Se decreases, the required sample size increases. If, however, the test Sp is also less than 100%, sampling more animals decreases the herd Sp and it is even more likely that disease-free animals may, incorrectly, test positive. A common solution to this problem is to submit positive animals to a second diagnostic test to confirm the diagnosis. Only animals that test positive on both tests are declared diseased. Considerations when using and interpreting "imperfect" diagnostic tests are discussed in greater detail elsewhere.[1] This review demonstrates, using formulae described by Dohoo and colleagues 2009,[2] how the required sample size changes depending on statistical considerations, such as the required precision of the estimate, the expected variation in the estimate to be measured, the desired level of confidence, and power of the test. For the scenarios discussed in this review we assume perfect Se and Sp. Computer software and free online sample size calculators provide a more exact sample size and also adjust the sample size for diagnostic tests with imperfect test Se and Sp.[3,4] We also assume that the farmer and veterinarian have the time, money, facilities, and other resources available to complete this investigation and that the farmer has a complete list of all animals (or sampling units), in the target population along with their unique identification number and other animal characteristics, such as age, sex, and parity as appropriate for each case study.

Epidemiologic studies may be either descriptive or analytical. Descriptive studies are commonly used to estimate a population parameter, such as a proportion or mean. For the veterinarian in clinical practice the population of interest is most likely to be animals within a farm, whereas veterinarians in government practice may investigate a "population" of regions within a country, or farms within a region. Descriptive studies may be used to determine the presence, absence, or prevalence of a disease or to measure production performance, such as the mean weaning weight of beef calves, or the mean somatic cell counts of dairy cows, in a population of animals. Often, the purpose of prevalence and "freedom from disease" studies is to support trade and the movement of animals at local, interstate, and international levels.[5] This may simply be a matter of testing the entire consignment of animals at a single point in time. For example, the veterinarian may be required to test rams for the presence of ovine brucellosis before introducing them to a new farm. Sometimes, however, certification requires evidence that the herd of origin is free of the disease. Sampling the entire herd is often not feasible. The challenge, therefore, is selecting an appropriate sample from the herd. Sampling strategies differ depending on the desired outcome, a disease prevalence estimate or certification of freedom from disease, and if there is clustering of the outcome within the population. Different sampling strategies for descriptive studies are discussed using case studies related to enzootic bovine leucosis in dairy cattle (Case Study 1), Q fever in goats (Case Study 2), and *Salmonella* prevalence in feedlot cattle (Case Study 3). Analytical studies aim to test associations between outcomes and exposures and may be conducted at a herd, farm, or regional level to support management decisions or to assess risk factors associated with disease or poor production performance. For example, the veterinarian may be required to measure the effect of different management strategies, such as housing or nutrition, on the prevalence of disease or daily liveweight gain. Different disease sampling strategies for analytical studies are described in Case Study 4a, sampling to assess the difference in disease prevalence, and Case Study 4b, sampling to assess the difference in mean liveweight gain.

DESCRIPTIVE STUDIES
Case Study 1. Enzootic Bovine Leucosis: Sampling to Estimate the Prevalence of Disease in a Population

Background

Enzootic bovine leukosis is a disease caused by bovine leukemia virus (BLV), a retrovirus that is spread horizontally via virus-infected lymphocytes. Overt clinical signs are rare affecting 0.1% to 10% of infected individuals. Bovine leukemia virus may, however, predispose the animal to opportunistic pathogens that cause mastitis and hoof problems leading to suboptimal production. Infection with BLV is also a barrier to local and international trade in many jurisdictions. Reports indicate an increase in BLV prevalence in the United States.[6] A US herd-level study found that 94.2% of US dairy herds had at least one BLV antibody-positive cow in the herd. The within herd prevalence was between 0% and 96.9% with an average of 42.5%. The prevalence increased from 29.7% in first lactation cows to 58.9% for cows in their fourth or later lactation.[7] All cattle are susceptible to BLV. Infection can occur at any stage of life and may occur naturally at parturition. Infection with the virus is lifelong and gives rise to a persistent antibody response. However, it may take up to 16 weeks for antibodies to appear postinfection and maternally derived antibodies can take up to 7 months to disappear. Antibody detection is the preferred method of testing.[8] Your client is interested in exporting her prized dairy cows to Europe and wants to know the prevalence of BLV in her dairy herd of 4000 females older than 7 months of age.

The sampling frame is a list of all sampling units in the source population. The sampling unit is the basic element of the population to be sampled. If the aim of this project was to estimate, for example, the prevalence of BLV antibody-positive dairy herds in a region, the sampling unit would be the herd and the sampling frame would be a list of all dairy herds. In this case, the sampling frame lists all cattle on the farm more than 7 months of age, along with their unique identification, their age, and parity.

The sample size

Equation 1 is the formula for calculating the sample size to estimate a single proportion.

$$n = \frac{Z_{\alpha}^2 \times p \times (1-p)}{L^2} \qquad \text{Equation 1}$$

n is the sample size.

Z_{α} is the value from the standard normal distribution corresponding to the desired level of confidence. α, the type one error rate is equal to (1 – the level of confidence). Many studies choose a 95% confidence interval, therefore α, = 1 – 0.95 = 0.05 and $Z_{\alpha} = Z_{0.05} = 1.96$. If we want a different confidence interval of 99%, $Z_{\alpha} = Z_{0.01} = 2.58$, and the required sample size increases.

p is an estimate of the proportion of seropositive animals we expect to detect in the herd. It may seem counterintuitive to estimate the prevalence of a disease in the population when this is the whole point of the disease investigation. We know that disease, especially infectious disease, if it is present in the population, usually infects more than one animal. We can, therefore, make an estimate of p based on prior knowledge from experience, or from the published literature. If in doubt, err on the side of caution, and choose $p = 0.50$, because this generates the largest sample size. If the expected prevalence is close to 0 or 1, the required sample size is smaller.

$p \times (1-p)$ is the variance of a single proportion.

L is the precision of the estimate and is equal to half the desired length of the confidence interval and is also known as the margin of error. How precise does the prevalence estimate need to be to meet the objectives of the study? If all other statistical considerations are held constant a larger sample size is required for a precise estimate. This means that if we want a narrow confidence interval, the estimate ± 0.05, we need a larger sample size than if a wide confidence interval, the estimate ± 0.30, is acceptable. The required precision for the sample size calculation is often based on nonstatistical factors, such as the availability of time, money, and other resources.

For this scenario we estimate a prevalence, *p* of 0.50. We want our estimate to be precise, *L* is ± 0.10, with a level of confidence of 95% (Z_α = 1.96), so that the minimum number of animals to be tested is 97. Note, that in sample size calculations, the number is always rounded up to the nearest whole number.

$$n = \frac{1.96^2 \times 0.5 \times (1 - 0.5)}{0.1^2} = 96.04 = 97$$

The sample size is adjusted for small populations of less than 100 animals, according to Equation 2.

$$n = \frac{1}{^1/_n + ^1/_N} \qquad\qquad \text{Equation 2}$$

n is the new sample size for a small population size.
n is the original estimate of the required sample size.
N is the population size.

The sampling plan

The required number of animals is selected from the population using simple or systematic random sampling. Simple random sampling requires that every subject in the population has an equal probability of being selected. However, we know that older cows are more likely to test positive for BLV antibodies than younger cows.[7] To ensure that each parity is equally represented, the best approach is to divide the population into mutually exclusive strata based on parity. The number of animals in each stratum selected for testing is proportional to the size of the stratum. For example, if 25% of the population is greater than or equal to third parity, then the sample size for this stratum is 25% of the total number of samples required, or approximately 25 animals. Random selection of 25 cows from this age group may be as simple as drawing 25 cow numbers out of a hat.[9] More sophisticated methods include using random number generators in free online software (eg, EpiTools).[10]

Systematic random sampling is often used if a complete list of individual identification numbers is not available. In this case, approximately 100 cows, from 4000 cows, need to be sampled. The first step of systematic random sampling is to randomly select a cow for testing from the first 40 cows that enter the chute, then select every fortieth cow from the rest of the population until the required number of samples is collected. This approach can also be used within stratum.

Case Study 2. Q Fever: Sampling to Detect Disease or Confirm the Absence of Disease

Background

Q fever is a nonfoodborne zoonotic disease. Ruminant animals (cattle, sheep, and goats) are the primary reservoir of the causative agent, the obligate intracellular bacterium *Coxiella burnetii*, and are the source of most human infections.[11] Livestock species are generally asymptomatic; however, approximately 40% of infected humans develop clinical disease. A study in Italy found that in goat flocks, with at least one seropositive goat, the average within-flock seroprevalence was 18%.[12] Your client is worried about the health of his family and asked you to assess if his flock of 200 dairy goats, older than 6 months age, is positive for the disease.

The sampling frame for this study is a list of 200 uniquely identified goats.

The sample size

Statistical considerations for finite populations of less than 1000 animals are discussed using Equation 3.

$$n = \left(1 - \alpha^{1/D}\right) \times \left(N - \frac{D-1}{2}\right)$$ Equation 3

n is the required sample size.

α = (1 − the level of confidence). The level of confidence is a measure of the probability of detecting disease if it is present. To be 95% certain of detecting at least one seropositive animal if the disease is present in the herd, $\alpha = 1 - 95\% = 0.05$.

N is the population size.

D is the estimated number of diseased animals in the group. That is, D = *population size × the minimum expected prevalence*. Again, we are asked to predict the proportion of the population that we expect to be infected if the disease is present in the flock. Based on the published literature, we expect, if the disease is present, that 20% of the flock (ie, 40 goats) will be seropositive. We want to be 95% confident of detecting at least one positive animal if the disease is present in the flock.

$$n = \left(1 - 0.05^{1/40}\right) \times \left(200 - \frac{40-1}{2}\right) = 13.02$$

A simple, random sample of 14 goats is required to be 95% confident of detecting at least one seropositive animal if the seroprevalence of Q fever in the flock is at least 20%.

For a larger or infinite population of greater than 1000 animals, the sample size is calculated using Equation 4.

$$n = \frac{\ln\alpha}{\ln(1-p)}$$ Equation 4

where $\ln$ = the natural log.

$$\frac{\ln 0.05}{\ln(1 - 0.20)} = 13.4$$

Case Study 3. Salmonella in Feedlot Cattle: Cluster Sampling to Estimate Prevalence

In the previous two case studies we assumed the sampling units were independent from each other. However, in many cases, the disease status of animals in cohorts or clusters within the farm are dependent on the disease status of other individuals within the cluster. A cluster is a collection of individuals with one or more characteristics in common.[2] A group of weaned dairy heifers raised in the same pen is considered a cluster because individuals within the cluster are often more alike than heifers chosen randomly from the population. The extent to which characteristics, such as disease status, of individuals within the cluster are similar is measured by the intracluster correlation coefficient (ICC), a value between 0 and 1 (Equation 5).[13]

$$ICC \text{ or } \rho = \frac{\sigma_b^2}{\sigma_b^2 + \sigma_w^2}$$ Equation 5

σ_b^2 is the variance between clusters
σ_w^2 is the variance within clusters

If the ICC equals 1 the disease is perfectly clustered by cohort. That is, if one animal in the cluster is diseased, all animals in the cluster have the disease. If the ICC is equal to 0, there is no clustering by cohort and the risk of disease is the same in each cohort. Cluster sampling and multistage sampling are examples of sampling animals within groups. For cluster sampling all animals within the cluster are selected for testing. For multistage sampling, a sample of animals within each cluster are tested. A common example of a cluster in ruminant animal clinical practice is a pen of cattle in a feedlot.

Background
In a US feedlot study, 9.1% of individual animal fecal samples were positive for *Salmonella* and 35.6% of pens had at least one animal in the pen test positive.[14] Another study in the United States reported a pen level ICC of 30%.[15] The manager of a feedlot in your practice is concerned about the safety of the meat from his farm and has asked you to conduct a study to estimate the prevalence of *Salmonella* positive animals in the feedlot. The feedlot has, on average, 10,000 animals, 50 pens of 200 cattle, on feed at any one time. You decide to conduct a diagnostic investigation to estimate the feedlot's prevalence of *Salmonella* positive cattle using a multistage sampling plan.

The sample size
Use Equation 1 to calculate a sample size that assumes independent data. If $Z_{0.05} = 1.96$, $p = 0.40$ and $L = 0.10$, the estimated sample size is 93. We then adjust the sample size to account for clustering using Equation 6. The final sample size not only depends on the ICC but also the number of animals sampled within each cluster. For this example, we start our calculations with a sample of 10 animals from each pen.

$$n = n \times (1 + \rho(m - 1))$$ Equation 6

n is the new sample size.
n is the original sample size = 93.
ρ is the ICC = 0.30. This is another parameter that is difficult to estimate and may not always be available in the published literature. The investigator needs to draw on knowledge of the disease dynamics to estimate the ICC.
m is the number of animals sampled per pen = 10.
$93 \times (1 + 0.3(10 - 1)) = 344.1$

The sampling plan
If 10 animals are sampled from each pen, a simple random sample of 35 pens (345/10 = 34.5) is drawn from the sampling frame of all pens in the feedlot. Ten animals are then randomly selected from each of these pens. If 20, 50, or 100 animals are sampled from each pen, the required number of pens decreases but the total number of samples increases (**Table 1**).

Table 1 Relationship between the number of animals sampled per pen, and the number of pens to sample and the total sample size[a]		
Animals Sampled Per Pen (n)	Total Sample Size	Pens to Sample (n)
10	345	35
20	624	32
50	1488	30
100	2856	29

[a] As the number of animals sampled per pen increases, the number of pens to sample decreases but the total sample size increases.

Choosing the appropriate number of clusters to sample and the number of animals to sample within each cluster depends on the relative cost of sampling individuals versus the cost of sampling clusters.[2] For example, if a farm is considered a cluster, the costs of driving to many different farms might outweigh the cost of sampling more individuals. Online calculators[4] consider the variability within and between clusters and the costs of sampling clusters versus sampling units to provide the most cost-effective sampling strategy.

ANALYTICAL STUDIES
Case Study 4a and 4b. The Association Between Management Factors on the Prevalence of a Disease and Production Performance

Background
Clinical veterinarians may be asked to assess the effect of different management practices, such as housing, diet, or vaccinations, on production performance or on the prevalence of a disease in the population. Production losses including mortality and reduced weight gain are frequently associated with respiratory disease in livestock. Loss of income is also associated with condemnation of consolidated and pleuritic lungs. Studies in New Zealand found that 28% of lambs had pneumonic lesions at slaughter[16] and that lamb liveweight was reduced by 1 kg/mo for every 10% of lung surface area affected.[17] A study in Spain found that even among lambs without clinical disease, 34% of lungs were condemned at slaughter because of the presence of pathologic lesions.[18] Respiratory disease is also associated with reduced liveweight gain in livestock. A sheep farmer in your area wants to assess if a newly developed vaccine against respiratory disease in sheep is effective in reducing lung lesions in lambs at slaughter and increasing the average daily liveweight gain of his lambs. The sheep farm produces 1000 lambs per year.

Case Study 4a. Respiratory Disease: Sampling to Assess the Effect of Vaccination on the Proportion of Lambs with Lung Lesions Detected at Slaughter

To calculate the sample size, the investigator needs to estimate the minimum desired effect of the management intervention. In this example the proportion of lambs with lung lesions at slaughter is currently 30%. The farmer has done some calculations and found that, accounting for the costs of the vaccination and the labor required to administer the vaccine, the proportion of lambs with lung lesions needs to decrease to 10% to break even on costs. Equation 7 is the formula for calculating the sample size for each treatment group to compare the effect of a treatment on the prevalence of disease in two independent groups.

$$n = \frac{\left[Z_\alpha\sqrt{2pq}+Z_\beta\sqrt{p_1 q_1 + p_2 q_2}\right]^2}{(p_1-p_2)^2}$$

Equation 7

n is the sample size
p_1 is the expected prevalence of lung lesions in unvaccinated lambs = 0.30
$q_1 = 1 - p_1 = 0.70$
p_2 is the expected prevalence of lung lesions in vaccinated lambs = 0.10
$q_2 = 1 - p_2 = 0.90$
p is the pooled prevalence$=\frac{p_1+p_2}{2}=\frac{0.3+0.1}{2}=0.2$ To detect a smaller difference in prevalence between the two treatments the sample size needs to be larger.
$q = 1 - p = 1 - 0.2 = 0.8$
$Z_\alpha = Z_{0.05} = 1.96$
Z_β is the value from the standard normal distribution corresponding to the power of the test. Power is the probability of detecting a difference if a difference truly exists. In many epidemiologic studies the required power is 80%. If the power is 80%, $Z_\beta = 0.84$. As power increases, so does the sample size.

$$n = \frac{\left[1.96 \times \sqrt{2 \times 0.2 \times 0.8} + 0.84 \times \sqrt{0.3 \times 0.7 + 0.1 \times 0.9}\right]^2}{(0.3 - 0.1)^2} = 61.5$$

Therefore, if the vaccine truly reduces lung lesions from 30% to 10%, then the lungs of 62 lambs, randomly selected from each group, need to be examined at slaughter to have an 80% chance of correctly determining that the new respiratory vaccine is effective.

Case Study 4b. Respiratory Disease: Sampling to Assess the Effect of Vaccination on the Average Daily Weight Gain in Lambs

Background
The sheep farmer reports a current average daily weight gain (ADG) of 180 g/d. Again, based on the farmer's cost-benefit analysis, he would like to see the ADG improve to at least 200 g/d following vaccination. Equation 8 is the formula used to calculate the required number of lambs to sample from two independent treatment groups, assuming that the variance in ADG is the same in both cohorts.

$$n = 2 \times \left[\frac{(Z_\alpha+Z_\beta)^2 \times \sigma^2}{(\mu_1 - \mu_2)^2}\right]$$

Equation 8

μ_1 is the expected mean ADG in unvaccinated lambs = 180 g/d.
μ_2 is the expected mean ADG in vaccinated lambs = 200 g/d.
To detect smaller differences in ADG between the two treatment groups, the estimated sample size needs to be larger.
σ^2 is the expected variance in average daily gain in the population. The larger the variance the larger the sample size. Estimating the variance, σ^2 can seem challenging and it is not a value routinely reported in published studies. First, we estimate from the farmers previous records that the range of ADG for 95% of the lambs on this farm lies between 120 and 220 g/d. The 95% range encompasses approximately $4\sigma.^2$ Therefore, $\sigma = \frac{220-120}{4} = \frac{100}{4} = 25$, $\sigma^2 = 625$ g^2/d.

$$n = 2 \times \left[\frac{(1.96+0.84)^2 \times 625}{(180 - 200)^2}\right] = 24.5$$

A minimum of 25 lambs in each treatment group needs to be measured to assess if ADG is increased by at least 20 g/d in vaccinated versus unvaccinated sheep.

Sampling plan for case study 4a and 4b
At weaning 1000 uniquely identified lambs are weighed and grouped according to weaning weight and sex. To reduce confounding, the study population of 140 lambs is randomly selected from a group of lambs of approximately the same weight and the same sex. Then, using a random number generator each lamb in the study population is assigned to either the treatment (vaccination) or control (saline injection) cohort. To prevent bias the farmer, the person administering the treatment, and the person collecting the data do not know which cohort is receiving the treatment. The cohorts are housed separately, to minimize the protective effect of vaccinated animals on nonvaccinates, and then managed using standard farm protocols until the day of slaughter when all study animals are again weighed and examined.

TARGETED SAMPLING

For some disease investigations, the population of interest is restricted to a target population within the herd or flock. For example, sampling to detect the presence of bovine Johne's disease in a beef herd targets cows older than 36 months of age and those with low body condition scores.[19] Certification of freedom of infection for reproductive diseases, such as ovine brucellosis[20] and bovine genital campylobacteriosis,[21] requires testing of entire males only because females are transiently infected, whereas males are often lifelong carriers of the causative agent. Targeted disease surveillance is also used for rare or absent diseases, such as bovine spongiform encephalopathy (BSE). To maintain international trade, many countries continue to conduct surveillance for BSE, despite having no reported cases for decades. The World Organization for Animal Health's (WOAH) targeted transmissible spongiform encephalopathies surveillance plan is designed to allow the detection of at least one case of BSE per 50,000 adult cattle in the population at the 95% confidence level. This system is based on points awarded for different types of samples. For example, Australia is classified as negligible risk for BSE and to meet WOAH requirements needs to collect 150,000 points for its targeted surveillance program over a 7 year period.[22] Samples collected from cattle between 30 months and 9 years of age with clinical neurologic disease contribute the most points to the surveillance program. Samples collected from fallen or casualty slaughter cattle are awarded fewer points. Targeted disease surveillance requires testing of high-risk groups. This reduces the cost of surveillance and provides greater confidence in the results of studies designed to provide assurance of freedom from disease.

SUMMARY

Diagnostic investigations in animal populations that are based on clear, realistic objectives and thoughtful planning provide information that is used to promote trade or develop management plans to improve animal health and production. The development of realistic objectives should be based on the availability of resources, time and money, and the availability of infrastructure to support handling and sampling of animals. The sample size is therefore determined by these nonstatistical considerations, in addition to the statistical considerations discussed in this review. Selecting the correct number and type of animals or sampling units to test, examine, or measure is critical to answering the diagnostic question and assisting the farmer to meet their management priorities.

DISCLOSURE

The author has nothing to disclose.

REFERENCES

1. McKenna SL, Dohoo IR. Using and interpreting diagnostic tests. Vet Clin Food Anim Pract 2006;22(1):195–205.
2. Dohoo I, Martin W, Stryhn H. Sampling. In: McPike MS, editor. Veterinary epidemiologic research. VER Inc; 2009. p. 33–56, chap 2.
3. Dhand N, Khatkat M. Statulator: An online statistical calculator. 2014. https:// statulator.com/. Accessed July 05, 2022.
4. Sergeant Evan. Epitools Epidemiological Calculators. Ausvet. Website 2018. Available at: http://epitools.ausvet.com.au. Accessed July 15, 2022.
5. Sergeant E, Cameron A, Baldock C. Epidemiological problem solving. AusVet Animal Health Services; 2004.
6. Bartlett PC, Ruggiero VJ, Hutchinson HC, et al. Current developments in the epidemiology and control of enzootic bovine leukosis as caused by bovine leukemia virus. Pathogens 2020;9(12):1058. https://doi.org/10.3390/pathogens 9121058.
7. LaDronka RM, Ainsworth S, Wilkins MJ, et al. Prevalence of bovine leukemia virus antibodies in US dairy cattle. Vet Med Int 2018;5831278. https://doi.org/10.1155/ 2018/5831278.
8. World Organisation for Animal Health. Enzootic Bovine" Leucosis, In: OIE terrestrial manual, - 2018, WOAH, 1113- 1124, chap 3.4.9. Available at: https://www. woah.org/en/disease/enzootic-bovine-leukosis/. Accessed August 08, 2022.
9. Cannon R, Roe R. Livestock disease surveys: a field manual for veterinarians. Canberra: Australia Australian Gvt Publishing Service; 1982.
10. Sergeant E, Perkins N. Epidemiology for field veterinarians: an introduction. CABI; 2015.
11. Ma GC, Norris JM, Mathews KO, et al. New insights on the epidemiology of *Coxiella burnetii* in pet dogs and cats from New South Wales, Australia. Acta tropica 2020;205:105416.
12. Rizzo F, Vitale N, Ballardini M, et al. Q fever seroprevalence and risk factors in sheep and goats in northwest Italy. Prev Vet Med 2016;130:10–7.
13. Killip S, Mahfoud Z, Pearce K. What is an intracluster correlation coefficient? Crucial concepts for primary care researchers. The Ann Fam Med 2004;2(3): 204–8.
14. Dargatz DA, Kopral CA, Erdman MM, et al. Prevalence and antimicrobial resistance of *Salmonella* isolated from cattle feces in United States feedlots in 2011. Foodborne Pathog Dis 2016;13(9):483–9.
15. Levent G, Schlochtermeier A, Ives SE, et al. Population dynamics of *Salmonella enterica* within beef cattle cohorts followed from single-dose metaphylactic antibiotic treatment until slaughter. Appl Environ Microbiol 2019;85(23). https://doi. org/10.1128/AEM.01386-19.
16. McRae KM, Baird HJ, Dodds KG, et al. Incidence and heritability of ovine pneumonia, and the relationship with production traits in New Zealand sheep. Small Ruminant Res 2016;145:136–41.
17. Alley MR. The effect of chronic non-progressive pneumonia on weight gain of pasturefed lambs. New Zealand Vet J 1987;35(10):163–6.
18. Lacasta D, González JM, Navarro T, et al. Significance of respiratory diseases in the health management of sheep. Small Ruminant Res 2019;181:99–102.

19. Collins MT, Gardner IA, Garry FB, et al. Consensus recommendations on diagnostic testing for the detection of paratuberculosis in cattle in the United States. J Am Vet Med Assoc 2006;229(12):1912–9.
20. Ridler AL, West DM. Control of *Brucella ovis* infection in sheep. Vet Clin North Am Food Anim Pract 2011;27(1):61–6.
21. Silveira CdS, Fraga M, Giannitti F, et al. Diagnosis of bovine genital campylobacteriosis in South America. Front Vet Sci 2018;321.
22. [AHA] Animal Health Australia. Maintaining Australia's freedom from TSEs. Animal Health Australia. 2021. Available at: https://animalhealthaustralia.com.au/maintaining-australias-freedom-from-tses/. Accessed July 17, 2022.

Submitting High-Quality Clinical Pathology Samples for Best Results

Yvonne M. Wikander, DVM, MS, DACVP*

KEYWORDS

- Blood smear • Blood tube filling • Fluid and tissue cytology • Point-of-care testing
- Sample acquisition • Sample handling • Sample shipping • Venipuncture

KEY POINTS

- Blood, tissue, and fluid cytology evaluations are some of the most reliable and cost-effective diagnostics available when properly acquired, handled, prepared, and shipped.
- The reliability of results is directly related to the quality of the patient samples submitted.
- Evaluating a cytology or smear before submission ensures the samples submitted are of diagnostic quality, saving time and money.
- If point-of-care testing equipment is used, regular maintenance, calibration, and validation through a managed quality assurance program is essential to ensure that results are accurate and reliable.

INTRODUCTION

Healthy patients are productive patients. This includes working dogs, emotional support or service animals, working ranch horses, productive laying hens, breeding livestock, dairy cattle, or feeder animals. In the pursuit of animal health and welfare management, clinicians and owners must often juggle the cost of diagnostics to obtain a reliabe and accurate diagnosis versus the cost of treatment and follow-up. Clinical pathology (testing of blood and/or tissue/fluids) are efficient and cost-effective diagnostic options; given the width and breadth of data provided. Maximizing the potential utility of clinical pathology testing options is contingent on samples being both representative of the disorder/lesion, and of a suitable diagnostic yield.

As such, the goal is to obtain, and submit, high-quality representative samples with the highest diagnostic yield to provide reliable results with which the clinician can have confidence. Without that confidence, a presumptive diagnosis is shaky at best. Subpar samples result in vague pathology reports causing frustration for all parties—

Department of Veterinary Pathobiology, VERO Program, Texas A&M, School of Veterinary Medicine, WTAMU Campus, 3201 Russell Long Boulevard, Canyon, TX 79015, USA
* Diagnostic Clinical Pathologist, Texas Veterinary Medical Diagnostic Laboratory, WT Box 60818, Canyon, TX 79016.
E-mail address: yvonne.wikander@tvmdl.tamu.edu

Vet Clin Food Anim 39 (2023) 33–47
https://doi.org/10.1016/j.cvfa.2022.10.003
0749-0720/23/© 2022 Elsevier Inc. All rights reserved.
vetfood.theclinics.com

diagnostician, clinician, owner—and subpar treatment of the patient resulting in prolonged illness, decreased productivity, increased expense, and/or poorer prognoses. This in turn may result in an owner and/or clinician with a dim view of diagnostic sample submission, which leads to less submissions... and the cycle continues.

During patient assessment, the clinician determines which organs system(s) is/are affected using the patient signalment, medical history, clinical signs, and physical examination findings. Preliminary problem and differential diagnosis (ddx) lists are then developed, often used an acronym such as DAMNIT (Degenerative, Amonalous, Metabolic, Nutritional-Neoplatic, Inflammatory-Idiopathic-Iatrogenic, Toxin-Traumatic or VITAMIND (Vascular, Inflammatory, Toxin-Traumatic, Metabolic, Idiopathic-Iatrogenic, Nutritional-Neoplastic, Degenerative). Diagnostic testing can then be selected based on the problem/ddx list generated (**Table 1**). In those conditions in which complete blood count (CBC) and serum biochemical laboratory tests would be enlightening, the specific tests selected can be based on the presumed organ system(s) impacted by the disorder or disease process to be ruled out and/or monitored (**Table 2**).

Once diagnostic test selection is determined, the clinician must determine what will be the *best* representative sample to obtain and then obtain those samples in a way that will optimize their diagnostic quality. The following is not a comprehensive how-to, rather a commonsense approach of "dos and don'ts" to optimize the sample(s) submitted to a clinical pathology reference laboratory or run using the practitioner's in-house laboratory equipment.

TISSUE CYTOLOGY SAMPLES

All abnormal growths and/or organ parenchymal abnormalities can be evaluated via fine needle biopsy with cytologic evaluation. The goal of this procedure is to identify if the tissue sampled is "normal," hyperplastic, inflamed, or neoplastic (benign vs malignant).

To have a diagnostic sample, the submitted slide(s) must:

1. Be the appropriate tissue,
2. Have sufficient intact nucleated cellularity to conclude it is representative of the tissue sampled,

Table 1
Diagnostics by VITAMIND differential list

		CBC	Biochemistry	UA	Cytology	Other Laboratory	Imaging
V	Vascular	√				√	√
I	Inflammatory	√	√[a]	√[a]	√		
T	Toxin	√[a]	√[a]	√[a]		√	√
	Traumatic	√[a]	√[a]	√[a]			
A	Anomalous						√
M	Metabolic		√		√	√[a]	
I	Idiopathic Iatrogenic						
N	Nutritional	√[a]	√[a]	√[a]	√	√	√
	Neoplastic	√[a]	√[a]	√[a]			
D	Degenerative				√		√

[a] Testing that may provide evidence of organ system involvement.

Table 2
Tests commonly used to elucidate compromise to specific organ systems

Organ System	Analytes
Digestive	
Gastrointestinal	Total Protein, Albumen, Globulin Cholesterol, NEFAB$_9$ (Folate), B$_{12}$ (Cobalamin) Sodium, potassium, chloride Calcium, phosphates, magnesium
Hepatic	Total protein, albumen, globulin Glucose, cholesterol, triglycerides, NEFA, BHB AST, LDH, IDH/SDH, GMD/GLDH/GDH ALP, GGT Bilirubin, bile acids Fibrinogen, coagulation panel
Endocrine	Cortisol, ACTH Lymphocyte concentration
Hematopoietic	Hemogram, leukogram, thrombogram Total protein, albumin Bilirubin Antinuclear antibodies Coagulation panel, vWF, thromboelastography
Musculoskeletal	AST, LDH, CK
Renal-urinary	Urea, creatinine, USG, UPC Phosphates
Electrolyte-acid-base	Sodium, potassium, chloride, phosphates Bicarbonate, lactate, anion gap, blood gas
Reproductive	Estrogen, progesterone, LH, FSH
Respiratory	HCT/PCV, RBC concentration blood gas, bicarbonate

Abbreviations: ACTH, adrenocorticotrophic hormone; ALP, alkaline phosphatase; AST, aspartate aminotransferase; BHB, beta-hydroxybutyrate; CK, creatine kinase; FSH, follicle-stimulating hormone; GGT, gamma-glutamyl transferase; GMD/GDH/GLDH, glutamate dehydrogenase; HCT, hematocrit; IDH, isocitrate dehydrogenase; LDH, lactate dehydrogenase; LH, luteinizing hormone; NEFA, nonesterified fatty acids; PCV, packed cell volume; RBC, red blood cell; SDH, sorbitol dehydrogenase; UPC, urine protein to creatinine ratio; USG, urine specific gravity; vWF, vonWillebrand Factor.

3. Spread sufficiently to visualize individual cells and their internal structures, and
4. Have minimal cell disruption or rupture.

As such, evaluation of one of the sample slides before submission is recommended and will be discussed below. Although inadvertent aspiration of an incorrect sample tissue is unusual, it can and does occur on occasion.

Sample acquisition can be successfully accomplished using techniques dependent on the tissues and/or lesions sampled. Obtaining and submitting 4 to 6 slides for each lesion sampled is recommended for the best diagnostic yield. The step-by-step specifics to perform the sampling techniques below are described in many textbooks (see "Resources" section) and will not be covered in-depth here.

- *The woodpecker coring technique* using a 21–23-gauge needle, 36-in IV extension line, and 6 to 12 mL syringe *without* negative pressure is optimal in most tissue types. Making sure the needle is rapidly driven into the tissue at different angles to obtain sample from multiple planes provides the most diagnostic sample. This rapid stabbing-like motion to fill the needle core with tissue cells is called the woodpecker technique. Because negative pressure is not applied, fewer cells are ruptured using this technique. If larger bore needles are used, the sample with be too thick, whereas using smaller bore needles results in suboptimal numbers of ruptured cells.

- *The woodpecker aspirate technique* is performed using the same equipment as described above with approximately 1 mL of negative pressure applied *after* the needle has been introduced into the tissue of interest. Greater negative pressure results in increased numbers of ruptured cells while smaller syringes do not supply sufficient negative pressure to obtain a representative sample. As with the woodpecker coring technique, making sure the needle is rapidly driven into the tissue at different angles to obtain sample from multiple planes provides the most diagnostic sample. It is important to discontinue the negative pressure *before* removing the needle from the tissue to avoid aspirating the sample into the syringe, where it is lost. Because negative pressure is applied, more cells may be ruptured using this technique. As such, this technique is best reserved for those lesions that do not yield sufficient sample using the woodpecker coring technique.
- *Superficial lesion impression smears and scrapes* can provide valuable information about these lesions. Ulcerated dermal lesions have a layer of superficial material (serum, debris, and superficial bacteria), which *will not* provide valuable information regarding the underlying tissue. Therefore, cleaning off the superficial layer using a saline-soaked gauze sponge before obtaining the impression smear can be helpful to avoid a nondiagnostic report. Once cleaned, rubbing a saline-moistened cotton-tipped applicator or scraping the surface with a dull scalpel blade held perpendicularly to the tissue often provides very adequate samples. If a cotton-tipped applicator was used, then it is rolled, not rubbed, across a clean glass slide to deposit sample. Whereas, if a scalpel blade was used, its material is transferred to the slide before spreading it with another slide (see the squash technique below). That said, an aspirate sample is always preferable.
- *Excised tissue impression smears* can provide excellent diagnostic samples if the tissue is dabbed repeatedly with gauze or toweling until minimal blood and/or serum is oozing from the tissue before making touch preps. Excess fluid interferes with the cellularity of the sample as well as cell adhesion to the glass slide. If there is no excess blood or fluids on the slide, then no further sample spreading is necessary. If the touch preparation does not yield sufficient intact nucleated cellularity, then scraping the cut surface with a scalpel blade held perpendicular to the tissue surface and transferring the cells from the scalpel blade to the glass slide before smearing (see later discussion) is a good second option.

Sample handling and preparation can also make or break the diagnostic value of a sample. Whether a sample is obtained using the woodpecker coring, aspirate, or scrape technique, the squash preparation technique must be used to spread the cells into a monolayer to be read. Blow-n-go or starfish/squish-n-go samples often do not provide the pathologist with a readable monolayer. Blow-n-go samples (**Fig. 1**A) are those that have been rapidly expelled across a slide in variably sized droplets that are not spread (**Fig. 1**C and 1D). The result is thick droplets of multicellular layers that cannot be evaluated cytologically. Starfish/squish-n-go samples (**Fig. 1**B) are those that have been expelled onto a slide as a droplet and had another slide placed on top of it, which is immediately lifted off. Although this preparation form can provide

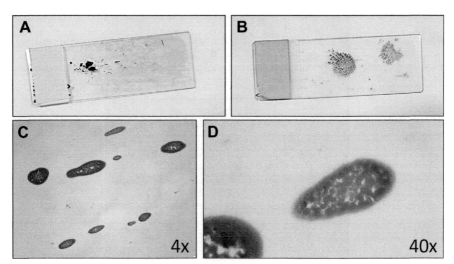

Fig. 1. Example of blow-n-go (*A*) and starfish/squish-n-go (*B*) samples. These samples have not been adequately spread resulting in thick droplets (*C* and *D*) without a monolayer to evaluate.

some areas with a monolayer, many of these samples do not have sufficient areas to be diagnostic samples.

For the squash (slide-over-slide) preparation technique to be successful:

1. Never ever clean and reuse slides.
2. The sample must be spread *immediately* after each slide production to avoid premature drying and cell rupture.
3. A light touch is necessary to avoid rupturing friable cells, especially lymph node preparations.
4. Once the sample has been transferred near the frosted end of a clean glass slide, a second clean glass slide is placed on top of the slide containing the sample but without downward pressure. The top slide is then drawn down the length of the bottom slide relatively quickly. Thus, spreading the sample with minimal cell rupture.

Evaluation before submission is recommended to ensure the sample is diagnostic. This will save time and money for all involved. To evaluate the sample, select one of the 4 to 6 slides obtained for staining. Neither select the best slide nor the worst, rather select one of quality in between. Staining with aqueous Romanowsky stains, for example, Differential Quik Stain Kits, should be accomplished using "clean" Copland jars; that is, jars that are *not* used for "dirty" samples, for example, feces or ear samples. Stain the slide per stain manufacturer recommendations and allow to air dry. Do *not* heat fix, use compressed air, or blow dry the sample because it can be damaged by heat and/or blown off the slide. Using a microscope, evaluate the slide sample to ensure it has numerous, intact, nucleated cells spread in a monolayer (**Fig. 2**). If not, take more fine needle biopsy samples following the above recommended steps to assess their diagnostic potential. If a diagnostic cytologic sample cannot be obtained, then tissue biopsy for histopathology may be more diagnostic. Alternatively, the slides obtained can be submitted to see if any data can be gleaned from them. In the latter scenario, practitioner and client should be aware that the sample may not yield diagnostic information.

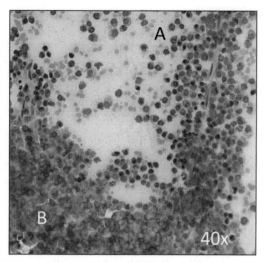

Fig. 2. A highly cellular sample. Evaluate a smear before submission to determine if there is a sufficiently cellular, well-spread, readable monolayer. This slide has both monolayer (A) and unreadable thick cellular areas (B). Note: a sample does not need to have the same level of cellularity depicted in this figure to be diagnostic.

Storage and shipment of cytologic samples have some important requirements to ensure the sample will be diagnostic. Send all slides inidvidually labelled within a box-like plastic or Styrofoam slide holder. Cardboard, thin plastic slide holders, and pill bottles are not sturdy enough for transport and often result in broken unreadable slides (**Fig. 3**).

Cytology slides cannot be exposed to *any* formalin in any form (fumes or fluid), because it fixes the cell membranes making them poorly permeable to stains (**Fig. 4**). As such, formalin jars should be stored far from the staining and packing stations and all cytology slides should be packed and shipped in an entirely separate box; *not* in a box within another box that contains a box of formalized samples.

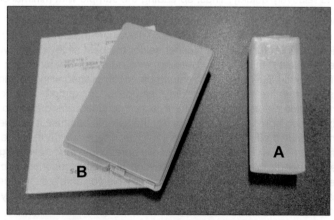

Fig. 3. To avoid slide breakage during shipment, use hard plastic (A) versus cardboard or thin plastic slide holders (B).

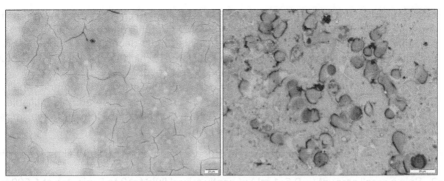

Fig. 4. Slides exposed to formalin fumes during shipping discolors the cells making internal structure evaluation impossible.

Submission forms should be filled out completely providing patient signalment, abnormal or unusual physical examination findings, pertinent history, clinician differential diagnosis list, and lesion location, size, appearance, and duration. If a skin lesion is being assessed, identify if it is in the dermis (moves with the skin) or in the subcutis (moves independently of the overlying skin). Pathologists are trained to correlate cytologic findings with the above history. If there is not enough information provided, then only vague conclusions can be made. Conversely, if the information provided consists of many unrelated details, then the sample results may be delayed due to the additional time needed to sift through the records provided and/or call the clinician for clarification.

Cytology limitations do exist and should be kept in mind when considering submission of a lesion sample:

1. Inflammation confounds cytologic features of many cell types making differentiation between benign and malignant changes challenging.
2. Because tissue architecture is not available for assessment with cytology preparations, determinations of malignancy/invasiveness can be challenging in many tissues.
3. Well-differentiated neoplasms cannot reliably be differentiated from "normal" or hyperplastic cell populations.

FLUID CYTOLOGY SAMPLES

Fluid samples could include body cavity fluids (abdominal, thoracic, pericardial), joints, cerebrospinal fluid (CSF; lumbar or atlanto-occipital locations), bronchoalveolar lavage (BAL), transtracheal wash (TTW), uterine wash, bile, urine, milk, abscess, or cystic fluid. All these fluids/effusions can be evaluated via cytology. As with most cytology samples, the goal of this procedure is to identify if the fluid sampled is "normal" or contains hyperplastic, inflamed, or neoplastic (benign vs malignant) cells and what pathologic process(es) produced it, did not allow for its removal, or if it originated from an external source. Fluid analysis can provide valuable clues as to its cause but rarely identifies the specific cause of its formation.

Detailed steps on how and where to perform fluid acquisition can be found in many texts and will not be covered here (see "Resources" section below). If there is sufficient fluid (>1 mL), all samples (see *Exceptions* below) submitted should have an aliquot placed in, (1) an ethylenediaminetetraacetic acid (EDTA; purple-top) tube for nucleated cell preservation, (2) a red-top tube (no preservative added) for possible biochemistry testing (bile acids, creatinine, glucose, lactate, potassium, triglycerides), and (3) a sterile tube for culture (anerobic/aerobic bacterial and/or fungal). If there is not sufficient fluid for the above, then the clinician must decide which portion(s) is/ are most important based on clinical impression of which would be most helpful with each case; generally, cytologic evaluation and culture.

Body fluids are harsh environments for cells and cause them to degrade rapidly. Cells sitting in fluids for as little as 24 to 48 hours are often rendered unidentifiable.[1] Therefore, the clinician can perform several steps at their establishment to maximize the sample's diagnostic yield by doing the following:

1. Make two (2) nonconcentrated direct smears using either a blood film or squash technique,
2. Spin a small amount (~0.5–1 mL) of gently mixed fluid for 3 to 5 minutes at 1,500 to 2,000 rpm (450 g),[1]
3. Using a refractometer, determine the total protein content of the spun supernatant,
4. Make two (2) concentrated direct smears from the spun pellet using either the blood film or squash technique, and
5. Bloody fluids can, and should, be spun in a microhematocrit tube and the packed cell volume (PCV) and total protein determined.
6. Cavitary (pleural, peritoneal, pericardial) fluids can be run through benchtop hemotology analyzers for total nucleated cell counts (TNCC) as long the fluid is free of clots.

Exceptions: All CSF should be submitted in red-top tubes without added preservatives. Only step #1 should be performed with CSF *if* a sufficient volume is collected. Additionally, joint fluid tends to be too viscous without the addition of hyaluronic acid for successful processing. As such, none of the above six steps is recommended when submitting synovial fluids.

All samples should be transported from client property to clinic on cold packs or refrigerated to preserve cellular details and avoid microorganism overgrowth. Shipping samples (tubes and slides within Styrofoam or solid plastic holders) should be mailed *overnight* on cold packs for best (most diagnostic) results. Again, exposure to formalin or formalin fumes will render samples useless.

As previously stated, submission forms should be filled out completely (see above *Submission forms*). With fluid cytology samples, include the volume of fluid removed, volume of fluid submitted, initial color and character (turbidity), and measured PCV and/or total protein, if performed.

Fluid cytology, similar to tissue cytology, has important limitations:

1. Inflammation confounds cytologic features of many cell types making differentiation between benign and malignant changes challenging.
2. Balled up cells, particularly leukocytes, are difficult to differentiate and/or evaluate for abnormal cytomorphologic characteristics or intracellular organisms. This limitation is most often found in synovial fluids and BAL/TTW samples.
3. Cystic fluids are produced by tissue lining or mass-inducing cells and are generally of low diagnostic value by themselves because they contain minimal, if any, nucleated cells. Thus, submitting tissue aspirates of the cyst wall in conjunction with the cystic fluid will provide the best diagnostic yield.

BLOOD SAMPLES

Blood samples can be used to obtain a great deal of information using a wide variety of potential tests including, but not limited to, CBC (complete blood count), variable serum or plasma biochemistry panels assessing different organ systems, toxicology panels, nutritional panels, and so forth. The goal of these assessments is to identify the organ system(s) affected and determine the pathophysiologic mechanism(s) causing the abnormal or unexpected analyte data. This in turn provides supportive evidence for the practitioner to generate a prioritized problem list and differential diagnoses, determine additional testing for further characterization/diagnosis, develop a treatment plan, and/or monitor patient response to treatment.

Studies show that most blood sampling errors (up to 77%) occur at the veterinary practice before sample submission.[2] Although some of these errors are avoidable (poor venipuncture technique causing hemolysis, incorrect blood tube selection, mislabeling samples, inappropriate storage, or incorrect packing for shipping to the reference laboratory), others are not (biologic rhythms, environmental effects). Additionally, animals under the influence of catecholamines, some medications (glucocorticoids), or dietary/nutritional supplements can also produce analyte results that are difficult to interpret and apply to the clinical problem. Indeed, marked hemolysis, lipemia, and/or icterus can affect the specificity of many serum biochemistry analytes.

Drawing a representative, high-quality, diagnostic blood sample includes several components:

- *Venipuncture site* should be selected for the fastest, safest, and least traumatic collection. This is often the jugular or tail vein.
- *Venipuncture site cleanliness* is important to avoid contaminating the sample obtained and introducing superficial material into the patient. Clean water, wet wipes, and alcohol are all viable sources for venipuncture site cleaning.
- *Venipuncture versus catheter.* If the patient has a catheter placed, blood can be drawn from that site. However, if used, discard the first 6 mL of blood obtained to avoid sample dilution from flush, fluids, and/or residual drugs in the catheter.
- *Vacutainer versus needle-syringe.* Vacutainer blood collection is the preferred method of blood acquisition because it draws the blood directly from the vein into the sample tube with only one pass through the needle, thus minimizing hemolysis. If a needle-and-syringe technique is used, use a syringe size that will apply an appropriate negative pressure for blood collection. Too much pressure will collapse the vessel and lyse red blood cells (RBCs), resulting in a slow, high-difficulty blood draw with excessive platelet activation and clotting of the sample. Smaller animals (foals, calves, lambs, kids, crias) with a low blood pressure may benefit from the use of multiple 1-cc or 3-cc syringes for sample collection. No matter which collection method is used, the needle bore should be no smaller than 23-gauge to avoid hemolysis, which can compromise the results, and thus interpretation of several analytes.
- *Appropriate blood tube use.* It is advisable to refer to your reference laboratories recommendations for the blood tube(s) to be used for specific tests or panels as clot activators or gels can interfere with some analyte measurements.
- *Blood tube filling.* When filling blood tubes containing additives, for example, EDTA, citrate, fluoride, it is important to fill them to the indicated fill line. Overfilling will overwhelm the additive and partially negate the reason for their presence resulting in analyte errors. Alternatively, underfilling will cause an overrepresentation of the additives purpose resulting in analyte errors. The magnitude of the error is proportional to the level of overfilling or underfilling of the blood tube. When using the vacutainer sample collection method, the tube's negative pressure will draw the appropriate amount of blood into the tube without undue pressure. If the needle-and-syringe

technique is used, remove the blood tube stoppers and the needle from the syringe, before filling the tubes directly from the syringe. This minimized the trauma (lysis) of blood cells because they are not forced back through the needle at high pressure. The one exception is the citrated coagulation tube (light blue top). This tube must be filled precisely to the line indicated and has sufficient negative pressure to do so. Therefore, with this tube, one can impale the blue top stopper using an 18-gauge needle attached to the blood-filled syringe and allow the appropriate amount of blood to be drawn into the tube.

- *Blood tube filling order* is important to avoid contamination of one tube with another tube's additive, which can, and often will, skew the analyte measurements. Blood tube filling order should be (1) coagulation tube (blue top with sodium citrate additive), (2) serum tube (red or tiger top with or without a clot activator), or (3) heparin tube (green top with lithium or sodium heparin additive), (4) CBC tube (purple top with potassium EDTA additive), and (5) glucose tube (gray top with sodium fluoride additive).

Once the blood sample(s) has/have been obtained, the serum tube must sit for a minimum of 30 minutes, or until full clot formation, before centrifugation. Once spun down, the serum can be placed in a separate red top tube or left in the serum separator tube. One to 2 fresh, unstained, air-dried, and labeled blood smears should be sent to the reference laboratory along with the whole blood and serum samples, packaged in a hard plastic or styrofoam box (see **Fig. 3**). Blood is a living, liquid tissue with viable cells that continue to metabolize product throughout their journey to the reference laboratory. Because they age, their cytomorphologic features can change, even within a few hours. Separating blood cells from serum and keeping all samples refrigerated will minimize these changes. The slides produced shortly after acquisition contain the freshest cells for the pathologist to evaluate. This is particularly true if the blood samples are delayed during shipping.

The step-by-step specifics of producing a high-quality, diagnostic blood smear are described in many textbooks and will not be covered in-depth here (see "Resources" section below). That said, the following are important pointers to produce high-quality blood smears:

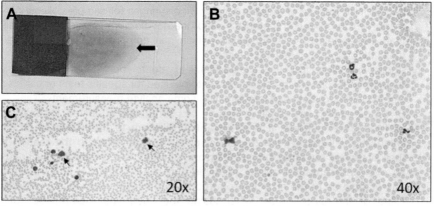

Fig. 5. Blood smear covering two-thirds of the slide (*A*) with a large counting window (*thick black arrow*). Note: internal structures of individual cells are visible (*B*) with minimal cell disruption or rupture. Ruptured cells are noted by small black arrows (*C*).

1. Never, ever clean and reuse slides for blood smears.
2. They should smoothly cover approximately one-half to two-thirds of the slide (**Fig. 5A**).
3. They should be spread sufficiently to provide a monolayer of RBCs, white blood cells, and platelets to enable visualization of individual cells and their internal structures (see **Fig. 5B**).
4. They should have minimal cell disruption or rupture (see **Fig. 5C**).
5. They must have a visible "counting window" (see **Fig. 5A** and B).
6. They should not contain choppy lines.

To ensure a high-quality smear has been produced, it is recommended to evaluate one of the sample slides before submission. Select one of the blood smears and stain it using an aqueous Romanowsky stain, for example, Differential Quik Stain Kits. This should be accomplished using "clean" Copland jars; that is jars that are *not* used for fecal or ear cytology samples, following the manufacturer's recommendations. Using a microscope, evaluate the slide sample to ensure it has readily visible, intact, nucleated cells (leukocytes) spread in a monolayer (counting window) (see **Fig. 5A** and B). If not, make several more blood smears taking care not to overstain them and assess their diagnostic potential.

As stated previously, all samples should be transported from client property to clinic on cold packs or refrigerated and labelled appropriately before being packed in appropriate shipping containers and mailed *overnight* on cold packs. Samples arriving more than 24 hours from collection time will likely contain artifactual changes often significant enough to question the validity of the results. Blood smears and tissue cytology samples that will be shipping in extreme cold can be fixed in clinic by dipping the slides in the methanol solution of an aqueous Romanowski staining kit (eg, Differential Quik Stain) for 15 to 20 seconds, air dry, and package in insulated containers to protect cell integrity, thus avoiding cell lysis in transit. Again, exposure of these samples to formalin or formalin fumes will render them useless.

Submission forms should be filled out completely (see above *Submission forms*).

POINT-OF-CARE TESTING–ACCURACY AND RELIABILITY ASSURANCE

Most practices are well equipped with a wide variety of in-house testing equipment. To be assured the results obtained from these items are accurate and reliable, the practitioner must control the quality of the results. As such, all practices should have a quality assurance (QA) program with written protocols for each piece of equipment ensuring regular maintenance, calibration, and some form of quality control (QC) monitoring. These steps ensure the equipment is reporting accurate and reliable results. This is particularly important for hematology and serum biochemistry analyzers, where calibration errors can cause large analyte errors, ultimately resulting in inappropriate medical decisions and adverse patient outcomes. A small calibration error in an analyte that is tightly regulated (calcium, creatinine, potassium) could be the difference between aggressive or conservative treatment, and therefore, life or death of the patient. Since the reliability of the test results is critical, regularly testing equipment for reliability is also critical. Imperfect results not only affect the success of patient care and outcomes but also affect second-order outcomes such as client satisfaction, practice growth and reputation, clinician income and job satisfaction, and practice staff's emotional well-being. Everybody wins with an established QA-QC program.

Equipment reliability is a factor of both its accuracy or bias (systematic bias error) and repeatability or precision (random error). Eliminating all error is unrealistic, so minimizing error to an acceptable range is the goal. These error ranges have been established to ensure that clinical interpretations and/or outcomes will not be adversely affected when they occur.[3] American Society for Veterinary Clinical Pathology (ASVCP) has published established "allowable error" for most analytes reported on hematology and serum biochemical reports.[4,5]

To minimize hematology and biochemistry equipment error, a QA program should: (1) include protocols to avoid preanalytical errors, (2) minimize interfering substances (lipemia, hemolysis, icterus), (3) use reference intervals representative of patient populations and locations served, and (4) use quality control material (QCM) regularly to ensure accurate (minimized systemic bias causing inaccuracy) and repeatable (minimized random error for improved precision) results are reported.[6,7] Unfortunately, the use of QCM is commonly omitted in practices due to its added cost and time.[7] This is problematic, as using QCM is the best way to maintain a determined level of accuracy and precision and, thus, a high level of patient care.

There are a few ways to minimize this cost but it is done at the expense of potentially missing equipment errors. Nonetheless, something is better than nothing. Cost minimization can be accomplished by the following:

1. Increase volume of point-of-care testing (POCT) to defray the per test cost of QCM. This requires a rigorous QC program stringently followed.
2. Only run *critical* bloodwork in-house. Charge appropriately to incorporate the cost of QCM, knowing it may price out testing to some, or many, clients.
3. Take an in-between stance. Run appropriately priced POC testing but spread out the use of a "normal" QCM. Generally, one should run controls (QCM) daily or with any change—the machine is turned on, calibrated, maintained, reagent changed, or suspicious patient results are seen. So, plan ahead. Leave the analyzer on for the whole week and run QCM once weekly when the analyzer is first turned on, for example, Monday start of business. Consider using only one level (normal) of QCM versus two. Arrange routine maintenance, repairs, and reagent changes to coincide with end of the week. If a change occurs within the week, then QCM should be run afterward to ensure the interactions are within acceptable error limits.
4. If a control run indicates the analyte results are inaccurate or unreliable, a series of steps must be taken before continued use of the equipment (**Fig. 6**).

The most cost-efficient way to manage a QC plan along with the above is to ensure staff are well-trained and document *everything*—policies, procedures, dates, times, who does what, when, where, and how. Confirm hematology results via blood smear review. Correlate analyzer hematocrits with spun PCVs. Consider forming a comparison group with other local area practices using the same equipment model. Every 6 to 12 months, each practice in the group runs the same blood sample on their analyzers, preferable around the same time of day. Each member is provided the data from all analyzers to make sure their results are similar. All analyzers are slightly different so it is unlikely they will all have the same results on any given blood sample.

There are 2 common myths regarding QCM that inhibit their use as part of the QC process in many practices.

Myth 1: Benchtop analyzers have internal controls making QCM unnecessary. Although analyzers do have internal instrument QC functions, they assess the internal electronic, photometric, and/or mechanical functioning of the equipment.[8] They do not assess the equipment, operator, reagents, and their interactions with whole blood and/or serum. The QCM is for the *external* QC of analyte analysis.[8] As such, a commercially available QCM recommended by the equipment manufacturer should be used.

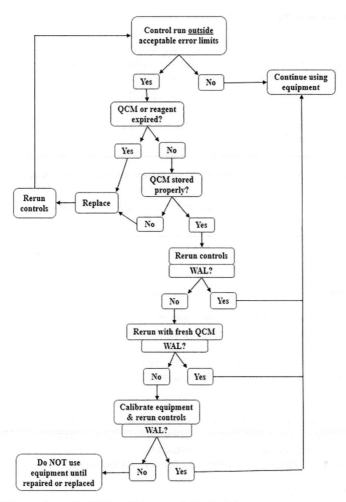

Fig. 6. QCM run schematic (WAL, within acceptable limits).

Myth 2: "Normal" patient blood and serum can be retained from one day to another and used repeatedly as a form of QC. Repeat patient testing-based quality control (RPT-QC) has indeed been evaluated and found to be acceptable for *dogs* using canine blood/serum, assuming the practice has access to normal canine blood daily.[9] However, this statement is somewhat misleading as a detailed process must be performed *before* using the RPT-QC system. The process includes obtaining pilot data from 20 normal canine samples and determining control limits for each analyte.[9] Without pilot data to use as a form of QCM, repeat testing of saved patient serum could vary widely from day to day as the sample slowly degrades. The author is not aware of any studies describing validation of RPT-QC for any ruminant species.

Unfortunately, following Myth 1 and/or Myth 2 practices makes the POCT results of questionable reliability and increases the risk of liability claims against the veterinary business and clinicians should a client bring suit. Formalizing a QA-QC approach to veterinary equipment only makes sense if the practitioner is going to make life-changing medical decisions for patients based on their results.

CLINICS CARE POINTS

- QA programs that ensure regular maintenance, calibration, and validation are essential to ensure accurate and reliable results from equipment.
- All practices should have a QA program to optimize the diagnostic quality of all their equipment.
- QCM use is a critical piece of a successful QA program, ensuring both accuracy and precision of equipment used.
- Perfection is unrealistic. The goal is to minimize error to an acceptable level.
- Do *not* rely on benchtop or penside POC equipment internal controls as evidence of good QC.
- If control run results are *outside* acceptable limits, *do not* use the equipment until it is replaced or repaired.

RESOURCES

Meyer DJ. The acquisition and management of cytology specimens. In Raskin RE, Meyer DJ. Canine and feline cytology: a color atlas and interpretation guide. 3rd edition. St. Louis: Elsevier, Inc; 2016. p. 1-12.

Meinkoth JH et al. Sample collection and preparation. In Valenciano AC, Cowell RL. Cowell and tyler's diagnostic cytology and hematology of the dog and cat. 4th edition. St. Louis; Elsevier, Inc; 2014. p. 1019.

VIN: https://www.vin.com/vin/

ASVCP Quality Assurance & Laboratory Standard Guidelines: https://www.asvcp.org/page/QALS_Guidelines?&hhsearchterms = %22qals_guidelines%22.

Westgard Rules: https://www.westgard.com/

Local clinical pathologist or veterinary reference laboratory.

ACKNOWLEDGMENTS

The author would like to thank those who provided insight into ruminant clinical practice including Lisa Lunn, DVM, BJ Newcomer, DVM, PhD, DACVIM, DACVPM (Texas A&M VERO Program Canyon, TX), and Jessie Monday, DVM, MS, DACVPM (TVMDL Canyon, TX). I am grateful to Julie Piccione, DVM, MS, DACVP (TVMDL College Station, TX) for providing photos of formalin-exposed cytology samples. Finally, I would like to thank Jessie Monday, DVM, MS, DACVPM (TVMDL Canyon, TX) for her brainstorming assistance.

CONFLICT OF INTEREST STATEMENT

The author declares no potential conflicts of interest or financial support with respect to the research, authorship, and/or publication of this article.

REFERENCES

1. Thompson CA, Rebar AH. Body Cavity Fluids. In: Raskin RE, Meyer DJ, editors. Canine and feline cytology a color atlas and interpretation guide. 3rd edition. St. Louis: Elsevier, Inc; 2016. p. 191–2.

2. Arnold J, Camus M, Freeman K, et al. ASVCP guidelines: principles of quality assurance and standards for veterinary clinical pathology (version 3.0). Vet Clin Pathol 2019;48:542–618.
3. Flatland B, Camus MS, Baral RM. Analytical quality goals—a review. Vet Clin Pathol 2018;47:527–38.
4. Harr KE, Flatland B, Nabity M, et al. ASVCP guidelines: allowable total error guidelines for biochemistry. Vet Clin Pathol 2013;42:424–36.
5. Nabity M, Harr KE, Camus MS, et al. ASVCP guidelines: allowable total error hematology. Vet Clin Pathol 2018;47:9–21.
6. Gunn-Christie RG, Flatland B, Friedrichs KR, et al. ASVCP quality assurance guidelines: control of preanalytical, analytical, and postanalytical factors for urinalysis, cytology, and clinical chemistry in veterinary laboratories. Vet Clin Pathol 2012;41:18–26.
7. Bell R, Harr K, Rishniw M, et al. Survey of point-of-care instrumentation, analysis, and quality assurance in veterinary practice. Vet Clin Pathol 2014;43:185–92.
8. Flatland B, Freeman KP, Vap LM, et al. ASVCP guidelines: quality assurance for point-of-care testing in veterinary medicine. Vet Clin Pathol 2013;42:405–23.
9. Flatland B, Freeman KP. Repeat patient testing-based quality control shows promise for use in veterinary biochemistry testing. Vet Clin Pathol 2020;49:590–606.

Metabolic Profiling in Ruminant Diagnostics

Robert J. Van Saun, DVM, MS, PhD, DACT, DACVIM (Nutrition)

KEYWORDS

- Metabolic profiles • Transition metabolism • Herd diagnostics • Metabolic disease
- Ruminant

KEY POINTS

- Animal selection for metabolic profile testing should be those not displaying clinical disease signs within designated animal groups of interest to answer a diagnostic question.
- Metabolic profiles provide herd-based diagnostics relative to disease risks and nutritional status based on appropriate animal selection and testing parameters.
- Use of metabolic profiling is best used to address animal performance, health, or reproductive issues associated with metabolic changes occurring during the transition period.
- Diagnostic success with a metabolic profile depends on proper sample collection and handling and having parity and stage of lactation blood analyte reference values.

INTRODUCTION

Measurement of blood components is a cornerstone of disease diagnostics in medical and veterinary practices.[1] Depending on the disease presentation, a clinician may order single or multiple analyte testing to complement the diagnostic process. Many clinical pathology laboratories offer specific blood analyte panels to address renal, liver, or musculoskeletal disease diagnostics; or more commonly a "complete" profile tailored to companion animal, horse, or ruminant animal disease diagnostics. Because our understanding of metabolism and associated physiologic changes associated with disease has expanded,[2–4] application of blood-based diagnostics has increased, with availability of newer technologies facilitating rapid and repeatable measurements of diagnostic analytes of interest. Newer immune response tests such as inflammatory cytokines and acute phase proteins (ie, haptoglobin, serum amyloid A) have been added to the blood diagnostic repertoire.[5] Use of blood analyte concentrations has traditionally been directed at disease diagnostics for an affected individual, and this perspective often confounds application to herd-based metabolic profiling.

The concept of metabolic profile testing (MPT) was first introduced by Jack Payne in Compton, England, in the 1970s and promoted as a method to differentiate metabolic

Department of Veterinary and Biomedical Sciences, College of Agricultural Sciences, Pennsylvania State University, 108 C Animal, Veterinary and Biomedical Sciences Building, University Park, PA 16802-3500, USA
E-mail address: rjv10@psu.edu

Vet Clin Food Anim 39 (2023) 49–71
https://doi.org/10.1016/j.cvfa.2022.10.004
0749-0720/23/© 2022 Elsevier Inc. All rights reserved.

superior cows.[6-8] Payne had suggested the selection for higher production brought on common metabolic diseases seen in the modern dairy cow; however, this concept can be applied to beef cattle[9,10] and small ruminants.[11-13] Metabolic profiling was developed for herd-based diagnostics rather than individual disease diagnostics, even though the Compton Metabolic Profile (CMP) was performed on individual blood samples.[6] Interpretation of findings from these samples was relative to calculated mean analyte separation ($\pm$2 standard deviations [SD], 95% confidence interval) from a defined population-based analyte reference mean.[7,8] This review will establish a rationale and practical methodology for applying MPT as a herd-based diagnostic or nutritional screening tool, as a component of evaluating disease risks of ruminant animals.

Defining a Metabolic Profile

A dictionary definition of a *metabolic profile* is an assessment of biochemical intermediates in tissues, which is used to describe metabolic pathways (https://medical-dictionary.thefreedictionary.com/metabolic+profiling).[14] Rowlands defined MPT as a "battery of tests run in concert to evaluate various aspects of metabolism."[15] A key component to the working definition for a metabolic profile is its application relative to animal numbers and selection. In contrast to using blood testing for disease diagnosis where one or more affected individuals are selected, MPT should only be applied to groups of animals that are not presenting with obvious clinical signs.[16] One could also select a group of "diseased" animals for comparison to unaffected animals as a part of a herd diagnostic process. Rationale for this selection process is to avoid confounding interpretation issues with disease-affected animals where physiologic responses would alter various blood analytes. For example, in response to an interleukin-1 inflammatory response, iron, zinc, and vitamin A will be sequestered reducing serum concentrations and serum copper concentration will increase due to hepatic release of ceruloplasmin, an acute phase protein.[17,18] Reduced iron and vitamin A concentrations can be observed due to suppressed hepatic synthesis of the respective transport proteins (eg, negative acute phase proteins).

As clinicians have relied on blood testing as a component of the collective diagnostic process, a similar perspective should be applied to MPT. More direct assessment methods such as animal evaluations (ie, physical examination, body condition scoring), records analysis, management practices (ie, grouping strategies, feeding program), environmental conditions (ie, heat stress, overcrowding), dietary evaluation (ie, nutrient content, particle size distribution, feed sorting), and facilities (ie, bunk space, watering units, heat abatement) assessment are all critical to herd diagnostics.[19-21] In contrast to past methods and typical current applications, MPT should be considered just one tool in the nutritional diagnostic toolbox. Results of an MPT should be used to direct or focus attention of a diagnostic process (screening tool) or to help confirm the presence of a herd disease process (diagnostic tool), although these are not mutually exclusive approaches.

Controversies

Blood chemistry diagnostics have been used since their inception for individual disease diagnostics. Application of blood chemistry diagnostics to ruminant metabolic profiling has been widely used and accepted in many countries.[22-26] In contrast, early applications of metabolic profiling in the United States suggested lack of diagnostic robustness with MPT relative to nutritional or health status assessment.[27-29] Additionally, perceived economic return on investment in an MPT was low due to high costs and low diagnostic outcomes, even though many laboratories had subsidized the testing.

A fundamental problem with the original CMP was animal group selection used to define superior metabolic performance. The process was intended to identify altered metabolism leading to "metabolic disease"; however, animal groups selected were not conducive to identifying this issue. Lactation groupings of peak milk and midlactation are more metabolically "stable" and would not reflect perturbations in homeostasis as it would in animals immediately following parturition.[30,31] Similarly, the CMP collected samples from dry cows collectively rather than recognizing, given more recent research, changes in nutrition and metabolism relative to time to parturition (eg, close-up vs far-off dry cows).[32–34]

Under controlled research conditions, blood analytes have been shown to be responsive to disease status, nutrition, immunologic response, and environmental factors (ie, heat stress).[35–41] Parity, milk production level, and days in milk were recognized as factors affecting blood analyte concentrations,[42,43] which accounts for the CMP group selection.[15] A wide range of factors beyond those of interest can influence blood analyte concentrations (**Box 1**). The animal selection process is used to minimize confounding variation. Sample[44] and animal[45] handling and laboratory-based concerns can be controlled leaving "environmental" factors that would reflect interherd differences.[46]

Diagnostic Rationale

Herd-level disease prevalence is a significant contributor to increased production costs and decreasing animal welfare. Transition of the ruminant animal from a pregnant, nonlactating state to a nonpregnant, lactating state is a metabolic challenge in maintaining homeostasis of critical metabolic substrates (eg, glucose, fatty acids, amino acids, calcium [Ca]), as well as other nutrients, leading to greater risk of periparturient disease conditions.[32,33,47] Modifications to substrate homeostasis in support of either pregnancy or lactation is under homeorhetic control.[48] A disease state is characterized by a critical alteration in metabolic processes, leading to specific clinical

---

Box 1
Factors contributing to variation in blood analyte concentrations

- Biologic variation
- Genetic variation
- Pregnancy status
- Season of year
- Circadian variation
- Production level
- Stage of lactation
- Parity
- Time of feeding
- Disease status
- Sample handling
- Laboratory analysis
- Environment
  - Herd of origin
  - Nutrition

signs of the disease. However, there is a spectrum of altered metabolism between a healthy (eg, no disease, good production, and efficient reproductive performance) and clinical disease state. We often consider a condition of altered animal performance without obvious clinical signs as "subclinical disease," such examples as subclinical hypocalcemia or hyperketonemia defined by specific ranges of Ca or beta-hydroxybutyrate (BHB) blood concentrations, respectively.[49,50]

Essentially, MPT should be used to define a "predisease condition" as opposed to blood diagnostics for a disease condition, especially on an individual basis. When one appreciates the complexity of metabolism and various influences from the environment, we can understand there may be one or more aberrations within the many body systems that may not result in a disease condition (eg, clinical signs) but would predispose the animal to impaired performance and risk for clinical disease. There have been multiple studies establishing statistical risk associations between serum nonesterified fatty acids (NEFA) and BHB concentrations relative to a specific disease (ie, left displaced abomasum, metritis, retained fetal membranes) or any disease event.[35,51–54] Testing for a single metabolic analyte ignores the interaction among various metabolic factors that may contribute to a disease state.[55] As an example, using mobilization of body protein in late gestation as assessed by 3-methyl histidine concentration, resulted in lower BHB concentrations early postpartum, suggesting amino acids are being used to stabilize glucose homeostasis.[56] However, if body protein was being extensively mobilized, then the cow presented with an excessive elevation of serum BHB concentration.[56] Similar metabolic interactions may also explain the lack of correlation between blood NEFA and BHB concentrations and how some individuals can maintain high NEFA concentration without declining into a ketotic state.[57] The diagnostic power of the metabolic profile is based on measuring multiple analytes to evaluate potential sources of metabolic disturbance rather than single analyte testing.

Blood Analytes of Interest to Metabolic Profiling

Measured analytes comprising an MPT tend to focus on energy and protein-related parameters and macrominerals (**Table 1**). Some laboratories allow for the submitting clinician to select analytes of interest based on their assessment of the clinical situation. Information from the University of Guelph Animal Health Laboratory emphasizes the need for the clinician to formulate a diagnostic plan with a hypothesis in planning the selection of analytes to be determined rather than just having a single profile template.[58]

Energy Analytes: Available energy to support maintenance and productive functions is considered a critical nutrient and one that most investigators have focused on relative to production disease conditions. Both NEFA and BHB have been considered the most useful blood analytes relative to disease risk while glucose, the key metabolic fuel, is often not considered useful diagnostically given its inherent homeostatic system.

- *Nonesterified fatty acids*—Products of adipose tissue lipolysis, which reflect the severity of negative energy balance. Serum concentrations are increased by low insulin and elevated cortisol and other adrenergic steroids. Serum concentration less than 0.25 mmol/L (mmol/L is equivalent to mEq/L [250 μmol/L]) are considered near neutral energy balance. Serum concentrations greater than 0.400 mmol/L (>400 μmol/L) or greater than 0.600 mmol/L (>600 μmol/L) are considered individual disease risk thresholds for late pregnant and early lactating dairy cows, respectively.[35,39,52,59] These concentrations are consistent across

Table 1
Blood analytes included in various metabolic profiles currently offered by veterinary diagnostic laboratories compared with the original Compton Metabolic Profile

	Analyte	Compton Profile	Michigan State	Oregon State	Guelph	TVMDL	Edinburgh	KSVDL
Energy analytes	Glucose	X		X	X	X	X	
	Triglycerides			X				
	NEFA		X	X	X	X	X	X
	β-Hydroxybutyrate		X	X	X	X	X	X
Protein status	Packed cell volume	X		X				
	Hemoglobin	X						
	Urea nitrogen (BUN)	X	X	X	X	X	X	
	Creatinine			X				
	Total protein	X		X	X	X	X (Globulin)	
	Albumin	X	X	X		X	X	
Liver function	Cholesterol			X				
	γ-Glutamyl transferase			X	X			
	Sorbitol dehydrogenase			X				
	Total bilirubin			X				
	AST			X	X			
Muscle protein turnover	AST		X					
	CK			X				
	3-methyl histidine							
Electrolytes, acid–base status	Calcium	X		X		X	X	X
	Phosphorus	X		X		X	X	X
	Magnesium	X		X		X		X
	Potassium	X		X		X		
	Sodium	X		X		X		
	Chloride			X		X		
	Anion gap			X				
	Total carbon dioxide			X				

(continued on next page)

Table 1
(continued)

Analyte	Compton Profile	Michigan State	Oregon State	Guelph	TVMDL	Edinburgh	KSVDL
Trace minerals							
Copper	X	O[a]		O[a]		X	
Iron	X	O		O			
Selenium		O		O		X (GSH-Px)	
Zinc		O		O			
Vitamins							
Vitamin A (total retinol)		O		O			
Vitamin E (α-tocopherol)		O		O			
Inflammatory analytes							
Haptoglobin				X			
Serum amyloid A (SAA)							

Abbreviations: KSVDL, Kansas State Veterinary Diagnostic Laboratory; TVMdL, Texas Veterinary Medicine Diagnostic Laboratory
[a] Optional testing available by the laboratory.

ruminant species. Serum NEFA concentrations are highest just before the first feeding.

- *Glucose*—Homeostatically controlled by insulin and glucagon. Contributions from hepatic gluconeogenesis from primarily propionate, amino acids, and lactic acid substrates. Low concentrations reflect a negative energy balance state while elevated concentrations may indicate loss of homeostatic control by insulin (eg, insulin resistance).[60,61]
- *β-Hydroxybutyrate*—The most stable of 3 ketone bodies generated by hepatocytes in the face of low blood insulin and glucose concentrations. Serum concentrations are considered the gold standard for defining state of hyperketonemia (Subclinical: >12 mg/dL [>1.2 mmol/L]; Clinical: >26 mg/dL [>2.6 mmol/L]).[62,63] Serum BHB concentrations are highest 3 to 4 hours following first primary meal as rumen conversion of microbial produced butyric acid generates dietary-sourced BHB.[37,64] Concentrations of milk or urine ketones can be useful diagnostically, although urine analysis is prone to false-positive test results, while milk can be fraught with false-negative test results.[39,65,66]

Protein Status Analytes: Next to energy, the availability of amino acids to support maintenance and productive functions has been the second nutrient of interest following energy.

- *Urea nitrogen*—It is sensitive to dietary protein status as influenced by dietary fermentable carbohydrate content and rumen solubility and degradability of the protein sources. Serum concentrations less than 8 mg/dL (< 2.85 mmol/L) would be of concern for inadequate protein, whereas concentrations greater than 16 mg/dL (>5.71 mmol/L) would be considered excessive for cattle. Higher values (>18 mg/dL [>6.43 mmol/L]) are normal in small ruminants. Creatinine is measured to assess potential for urinary filtration compromise influencing urea nitrogen concentrations.
- *Total protein*—It measures both albumin and globulins minus fibrinogen used to make the blood clot. Values can be altered by changing albumin and globulin concentrations confounding interpretation. Low values (<5 g/dL [< 50 g/L]) would suggest protein deficiency or loss, whereas high values (>8 g/dL [>80 g/L]) might indicate active immune response, dehydration, or both. A summary of protein fractions found in healthy cows have been published.[67,68] A plasma ratio of albumin-to-globulin may be an early indicator of inflammation and disease risk.[69]
- *Albumin*—The constitutive protein in blood responsible for maintaining osmotic pressure and important nonspecific transporter of minerals, fatty acids, and other molecules. It is synthesized in the liver and has a blood half-life of approximately 21 days. Considered a negative acute phase protein as in an inflammatory response, the liver will direct available amino acids for positive acute phase proteins in lieu of other constitutive negative acute phase proteins. Blood concentrations less than 2.0 g/dL (< 20 g/L) are considered indicative of protein malnutrition. Elevated concentrations (>5.0 g/dL [>50 g/L]) may be indicative of dehydration.[67,68]
- *Creatine kinase (CK)*—Specific leakage enzyme unique to striated muscle associated with muscle turnover. Laboratory reference range (95% confidence interval) is between 50 and 150 U/L for ruminants with some variation between laboratories. Excessively elevated values (>2000 U/L) are associated with severe muscle damage, although moderately elevated activities may suggest increased muscle turnover.

- *Aspartate aminotransferase (AST)*—Leakage enzyme due to cellular damage associated with either muscle cell or hepatocyte insults. Expected individual animal reference values range from 0 to 189 U/L for most ruminant species.

Liver Function Analytes: Ruminant animals seemingly are challenged while processing mobilized fatty acids in a state of negative energy balance. Multivariable blood analytes have been used to calculate different predictors of hepatic function relative to inflammatory response.[70–72] Hepatic lipidosis is a common sequelae or concurrent condition with many periparturient disease conditions.[73]

- *L-Iditol dehydrogenase*—This enzyme was formerly defined as sorbitol dehydrogenase.[1] An acute liver-specific leakage enzyme from damaged hepatocytes. This enzyme is more specific to ruminant species than other measured liver enzymes. Reference range is between 0 and 50 U/L for ruminant species with higher range for goats.
- *Glutamate dehydrogenase*—This is another hepatic mitochondrial leakage enzyme that indicates severe hepatocyte damage. Not all laboratories offer analysis for this enzyme, although this is a useful enzyme for large animals. Reference range is between 0 and 60 U/L with a lower range for alpacas (20 U/L).
- *γ-Glutamyl transferase*—An enzyme found in many organs, especially those with secretory function and is found in high concentrations in hepatocytes of ruminants compared with other species. Serum concentrations indicate potential hepatobiliary disease as the enzyme is released into blood following cellular damage. A laboratory reference range for individual ruminant animals is between 0 and 50 U/L with slightly higher upper level for sheep.
- *Total cholesterol*—Important sterol molecule relative to lipid transport and metabolism and substrate for synthesis of other steroid hormones (ie, vitamin D, estrogen, progesterone, testosterone). Serum total cholesterol declines in late gestation to a nadir (~70 mg/dL [1.81 mmol/L]) around the time of parturition, then increases to very high concentrations (>300 mg/dL [7.77 mmol/L]) into lactation. This pattern mimics feed intake thus cholesterol may provide some insight into intake. Cholesterol is often used to assess the liver's ability to export very low-density lipoprotein export. Calculating a NEFA:cholesterol ratio (mass ratio is unitless) has been suggested to assess fatty liver status.[74] Alarm values of greater than 0.15 and greater than 0.20 for dry and fresh cows, respectively, indicate potential hepatic fat infiltration risk.
- *AST*—Refer to protein evaluation above.
- *Total bilirubin*—Total bilirubin concentration in serum is a test of hepatic function.[1] Bilirubin is a pigment generated by the liver during breakdown of hemoglobin in red blood cells. Elevated total bilirubin (>0.5 mg/dL [>8.55 μmol/L]) is suggestive of impaired hepatic function. Normal serum concentrations range from 0 to 0.5 mg/dL [0–8.55 μmol/L] in most ruminants.

Electrolytes Status: Macrominerals, namely Ca, phosphorus (P), magnesium (Mg), potassium (K), sodium (Na), and chloride (Cl), play critical roles in muscle contraction, transmembrane electrical potentials, and acid–base balance, among other functions. Hypocalcemia has been a foundational metabolic disease of dairy cattle that has spurred much research as to underpinning mechanisms and methods of prevention.[75–79] Its association with many other postparturient diseases and immunologic function has led to it being described as a "gateway" disease in the transition dairy cow.[80–84]

Hypocalcemia and hypomagnesemia have received the most focus relative to serum concentrations and disease states. Macrominerals are homeostatically controlled to varying degrees and are thus considered to be of less diagnostic value. Low serum inorganic P is associated with hypocalcemia; however, a prolonged hypophosphatemia independent of hypocalcemia can result in a downer cow presentation.[85,86] In a retrospective study randomly selecting 30 cows from 2 transition feeding studies,[87,88] serum mineral concentrations during the 4 weeks before and following calving were determined and related to postpartum disease risk.[89,90] Health status or its interaction with prepartum or postpartum periods was significant for Ca, Na, Cl, and Mg (**Table 2**). Low prepartum serum concentrations of Ca (<8.0 mg/dL [< 2.0 mmol/L]) and Na (<133 mEq/L) were associated with a 3.8-times and 5.7-times greater risk for postpartum disease, respectively (**Table 3**). In contrast, elevated prepartum K (≥4.8 mEq/L) was associated with a 3.1-times greater risk for postpartum disease. Associations of serum mineral concentrations with specific disease conditions were also identified (**Table 4**). These data suggest serum macromineral concentrations are dynamic during the transition period and are useful diagnostically in MPT.

Trace Minerals and Vitamins: Trace minerals and fat-soluble vitamins are intimately associated with immune function and are physiologically altered in an inflammatory response. Although some serum trace mineral concentrations are not sensitive to nutritional changes (ie, copper, zinc), collection of multiple samples can assess herd-based differences.[91] Serum vitamins A, D, and E concentrations physiologically decline before calving due to losses to colostrum.[92] Low serum concentration of α-tocopherol has been associated with an increased risk of mastitis and retained placenta.[93,94] Increasing serum retinol concentration before calving has been associated with reduced postpartum mastitis risk.[94] Collectively, trace minerals and vitamins in their roles as antioxidants have implications for metabolic alterations during pregnancy and lactation.[95–97]

Immunity and Inflammatory Response Analytes: Recent research has focused on the role of an activated inflammatory response as the underpinning issue leading to periparturient diseases.[31,98–100] Haptoglobin, an acute phase protein, has been mostly investigated relative to disease risk.[101–103] Acute phase proteins and other biomarkers of inflammation are also being evaluated relative to disease risks.[71,72,104,105]

Application Methods

To obtain useful information from the data collected from blood analysis, one needs to focus on developing an initial diagnostic hypothesis and collect samples accordingly. The most critical aspect of performing a blood metabolic profile is appropriate animal selection.

- *Animal Selection*: In contrast to what most clinicians would do when performing blood diagnostics, animals that are not exhibiting outward clinical manifestations of disease should be selected for sampling. **Table 5** provides a suggested grouping of animals to be selected based on transition cow disease concerns.[19,51] Additional lactating groups or reproductive status groups can also be selected depending on the underlying problem being addressed. It is important to address parity and days in milk in sampling individuals between lactating groups.[15,43] Statistically, it has been suggested that 10 to 12 animals be selected per group, whereas the original CMP selected 7 animals per group.[7,20] Obviously, the more samples the better the assessment of the population but economics is the limiting factor.

Table 2
Comparison of least squared mean (± standard error) serum mineral concentrations in dairy cows that differed by documented health events (0 vs 1 or more) during the 4 weeks before and following calving

Mineral	Units	Prepartum		Postpartum		Effect P < F		
		Healthy	Sick	Healthy	Sick	Health	Period	H x P
Calcium	mg/dL	8.55 ± 0.16	8.10 ± 0.12	8.97 ± 0.16	8.15 ± 0.12	<.0001	.08	.18
	mmol/L	2.14 0.04	2.03 ± 0.03	2.24 ± 0.04	2.04 ± 0.03			
Sodium	mEq/L	140.3 ± 2.0	135.9 ± 1.4	142.0 ± 2.0	133.3 ± 1.4	.0004	NS	.19
Chloride	mEq/L	103.1 ± 0.5	102.2 ± 0.4	99.6 ± 0.5	98.6 ± 0.4	.05	<.0001	NS
Magnesium	mg/dL	2.19 ± 0.05	2.31 ± 0.04	2.47 ± 0.05	2.32 ± 0.04	NS	.0005	.0014
	mmol/L	0.90 ± 0.02	0.95 ± 0.02	1.02 ± 0.02	0.95 ± 0.02			

Cows were selected from 60 cows (21 healthy, 39 sick) with sick cows experiencing on average 1.9 health events (1–6 range).

[a] Covariate-adjusted means for effect of trial: Vallimont et al., 2001 and Ordway et al., 2002.

Table 3
Postpartum risk for any disease event based on mean serum mineral concentration in either the 4 weeks prepartum or postpartum in transition dairy cows (n = 60)

Mineral	Period	Threshold Criteria	Odds Ratio	95% Confidence Interval	P ≤ F
Calcium	Prepartum	< 8.0 mg/dL (<2.0 mmol/L)	3.8	1.2–12.4	0.02
	Postpartum	< 8.0 mg/dL (<2.0 mmol/L)	4.0	1.1–14.1	0.03
Potassium	Prepartum	≥ 4.8 mEq/L	3.1	1.1–9.3	0.04
Sodium	Prepartum	< 137 mEq/L	5.2	1.7–15.9	0.003
	Postpartum	< 137 mEq/L	8.3	2.5–27.8	0.0003

Postpartum mineral concentrations may reflect a consequence of the disease process.

- *Sample Collection*: The single most important aspect in sample collection is prevention of hemolysis. Serum is the desired sample for MPT because most laboratories have their reference values based on serum and not plasma. Hemolysis will adversely affect many analytes, thus confounding their interpretation.[44] The appropriate vacuum blood tube should be used for the desired sample (**Table 6**). Coccygeal blood is the preferred sampling site because jugular and mammary vein samples will have altered analyte concentrations due to metabolite extraction by salivary and mammary gland, respectively.[106] Timing of samples relative to feeding also is important but this will differ relative to the analyte of interest and can be accounted for in the interpretation.[20,64]

Table 4
Mean serum mineral concentration either during the 4 weeks before (pre) or following (post) calving in transition dairy cows compared between healthy (no disease events) and diagnosed disease conditions

Mineral	Healthy Cows n = 21		Mastitis n = 14		Retained Fetal Membranes n = 10		Ketosis n = 10		Udder Edema n = 15	
	Pre	Post	Pre	Post	Pre	Post	Pre	Post	Pre	Post
Ca, mg/dl	8.48	8.86			7.77	7.88	8.25	8.03	7.99	8.25
Ca, mmol/L	2.12	2.22			1.94	1.97	2.06	2.01	2.00	2.06
Mg, mg/dl	2.23	2.48		2.24				2.34		2.39
Mg, mmol/L	0.92	1.02		0.92				0.96		0.98
Na, mEq/L	140.5	141.1			135.4	131.9	132.9	128.1	135.9	133.5
Cl, mEq/L	103.1	101.5	99.7	98.5			102.1	98.6	102.2	98.2
K, mEq/L	4.57	4.88							4.83	4.95
Fe, µg/dL	181	149	218	162						
Fe, µmol/L	32.4	26.7	39.0	29.0						
Zn, µg/dL	1.12	0.93			1.07	0.87				
Zn, µmol/L	17.13	14.22			16.37	13.31				

Cows may have had more than one of the diseases. All mean comparisons within period (pre vs post) by disease condition are significant at $P < .05$.[a]

[a] Disease definitions: Mastitis = somatic cell count > 200,000, abnormal milk secretion with udder redness, or a combination; Retained fetal membranes = retained > 24 h after calving; Ketosis = observed signs of off feed, reduced milk production, and positive urine ketostix test; Udder edema = any pitting edema to teat and/or udder.

Table 5
Organization of sample collection for metabolic profiling

Physiologic Groups	Time Relative to Calving	Parity	Disease Status
Far-off dry	>10 d following dry off and <30 before calving	Keep heifers and 2+ lactation animals separate—pool as separate parity groups within physiologic groups	Unknown
Close-up dry	Between 3 and 21 d before calving (3–14 d best)		Unknown
Fresh	3–30 d in milk (7–21 d best)		Group cows with and without disease within lactational groups—keep days in milk similar within and between groups
Lactation groups	Define as needed based on disease conditions, production level or other problem		

- *Interpretation of Results*: Interpretation critically depends on appropriate reference values for the metabolites of interest accounting for variation due to parity and time relative to parturition. Many diagnostic laboratories have population 95% reference ranges for blood analytes but these may not be adjusted for time relative to parturition or age. Recently published studies have provided suggested reference values for cattle during the transition period.[58,67,107–109]
  - *Individual samples:* Blood analyte results would be compared with laboratory reference values in considering a clinical disease issue but more importantly, in MPT, they would be compared with a defined threshold value associated with an increased disease risk.[110] Interpretation is based on the percentage of samples above or below the defined critical threshold associated with disease risk.[46,111–115] Herd alarm levels for NEFA and BHB concentrations for disease risk at 15% showed impaired cow performance.[113] Others have made general recommendations of 20% to 25% of cases to be of concern in herd testing.[112,114]
  - *Mean or Pooled samples*: The CMP measured blood analyte concentrations in individual samples (21 in total; 7 per 3 groups) then calculated the mean analyte concentration and compared with a herd-based analyte value.[7,8] Calculated mean values were interpreted as abnormal if they deviated more than 2 SD from the defined population mean. This approach allows for investigation of individual variation within samples but comes with a high cost for testing. Others have questioned the simplistic approach of using 2 SD for all analytes given the wide range of variation across blood analytes.[27,116]

The use of pooled samples in lieu of calculated means has been proposed to reduce incurred costs of MPT.[117] Pooling samples is easily accomplished by pipetting an equal amount of serum (25–100 μL depending on number of samples) from individuals to be included in the final sample. Most laboratories require a minimum of 0.5 mL sera to complete an extensive chemistry panel. Check with the laboratory for the required volume to complete all desired testing. Mixing of serum has not resulted in clotting or any abnormal reactions that affect testing procedures. Based on the author's experience, suggested pooled sample size is best between 5 and 15 individuals. If more

Table 6
Blood collection tubes and their purpose relative to metabolic profiling

Stopper Color	Additive	Sample Obtained	Intended Use/Disadvantages
Red	None	Serum	Routine use for all metabolic profiles. Prolonged clot exposure results in ↓ glucose, Ca and ↑ phosphorus. Hemolysis problems in poorly handled samples
Red "Tiger" stripe or yellow	Polymer gel and silica clot activator	Serum	Serum separator tube. Routine for all tests. Clot separation is often not complete leading to hemolysis or red blood cell contamination. Should *not* be used for metabolic profiles
Gray	Na fluoride or K oxalate	Serum	Glycolytic Inhibitor for sensitive glucose analysis—not appropriate for other analyses within metabolic profiles
Royal blue	Plastic stopper ± Na heparin	Serum or plasma	Trace mineral analysis—especially for zinc. Serum samples preferred for metabolic profiles
Lavender	Ethylenediaminetetraacetic acid (EDTA)	Whole blood Plasma	Routine use for complete blood count/ EDTA chelates Ca, Mg and ↓ enzyme activities. Should *not* be used for metabolic profiles
Green	Na Heparin	Plasma Whole blood	Routine analyses for either plasma or whole blood/no effect on metabolites. Could be used for metabolic profiles if laboratory has reference values for plasma rather than serum

individuals are available, it might be best to make multiple pools to gain some variability assessment. Measured analyte concentrations in a pooled sample are not different from calculated means.[104,117–121] Interpretation of pooled samples should be performed relative to deviation from herd-based population means or medians with the SD similar to the original concept of the CMP. The following methods have been used to interpret pooled samples:

1. Number of SD from a defined population reference value. Analytes with low variation (ie, Ca, glucose, Na, Mg) may have significant alterations at only 0.5 SD difference. Analytes with moderate variation (ie, BHB, NEFA, Blood urea nitrogen [BUN], P, cholesterol) might vary by 0.5 to 1 SD from reference mean. Analytes with high variation (ie, CK, liver enzymes) would need to deviate by 1.5 or more SD.
2. Define a lower threshold value for an analyte relative to what has been documented for an individual animal to be associated with greater risk for disease or impaired animal performance.[118]
3. Use of statistical process control charts to monitor changes in analyte means over time.[122]

What is critical to interpretation is the herd-based reference values and animal selection where no clinical disease animals are included that could skew the pooled value. In preliminary study by the author, a positive linear relationship between percent of abnormal analyte values within a pool (based on individual sampling) and number of

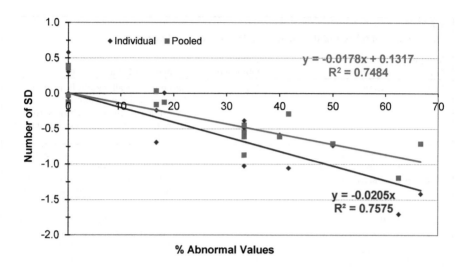

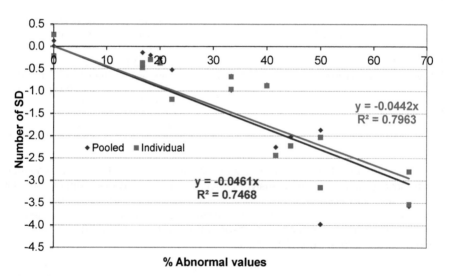

Fig. 1. Plot of the number of SD a sample deviates from a defined healthy population mean value for (*A*) NEFA (0.43 ± 0.31 mEq/L) and (*B*) β-hydroxybutyrate (8.1 ± 3.2 mg/dL) relative to percent of abnormal individual values within the sample in fresh dairy cows. Individual sample result was a calculated mean of individual test results. Percent abnormal values was determined by the number of individual samples exceeding a defined threshold for NEFA (>.6 mEq/L) and BHB (>1.0 mmol/L). Sample number within a pool ranged from 5 to 12 individuals.

SD the sample mean was from the reference mean (**Fig. 1**). Based on the Ospina work[52,113] targeting 15% to 20% abnormal values, one could determine the critical number of SD for each analyte measured for pooled samples.

Current Evidence

As stated, application of MPT was well received outside of the United States. Since publication of the Ingraham and Kappel review of MPT,[123] there were infrequent North

American publications addressing MPT. Since the early 2000s there seemed to be renewed interest in MPT in dairy herds most likely the result of increasing dairy herd size.[16] Increasing herd size can address the economic issues given the potential return on investment if a herd-wide issue is adequately identified and corrected. In concert with herd size, research has continued to provide further understanding of metabolic alterations associated with animal health and performance. A simple Google Scholar search for "metabolic profiling dairy cattle" provides more than 30,000 publications with most being published since 2000. Although pooled sample studies are limited,[104,118,119] there is much interest and application of pooled samples relative to infectious and parasitic disease and nutritional diagnostics.

FUTURE DIRECTIONS

Research continues to develop new and improved diagnostic aids for herd disease risk, nutritional status, and reproductive performance assessment. Much interest is in the use of milk as a vehicle for analyte measures because this would be a more convenient sample.[124,125] Novel on-farm testing for NEFA and BHB as well as use of Fourier-transform infrared spectroscopy or nuclear magnetic resonance are tools being developed.[126–130] Alternative metabolites are being recognized as better disease, reproduction, or productive predictors.[131–135] Newer statistical methods are being used to identify metabolite groups or clusters associated with disease risk.[124,136,137] The greatest expansion of transition cow metabolism has been applying the fields of proteomics and metabolomics.[138–141] These areas will continue to expand our knowledge and diagnostic capabilities in the effort to reduce disease risk and identify disease risk in a more timely fashion.

CLINICS CARE POINTS

- Metabolic profiling in the strictest sense of the application is a herd-based screening diagnostic tool to be used in concert with other direct diagnostic methods (ie, production and health records analysis, animal evaluations, dietary assessment).

- Performing a herd metabolic profile should be a defined diagnostic investigation intending to collect data relative to a specific question or hypothesis.

- A metabolic profile should be performed on animals not exhibiting obvious clinical signs as opposed to a disease diagnosis of clinically affected animals. Comparisons between affected and unaffected animals may be used to potentially define underlying metabolic differences that may underpin the disease process.

- Pooling of samples within specified animal grouping may provide the best return on investment although improvements are needed in better defining interpretation.

DISCLOSURE

Grant funding received from Pennsylvania Department of Agriculture, United States, American Dairy Goat Association, United States, Zoetis, United States.

REFERENCES

1. Russell KE, Roussel AJ. Evaluation of the ruminant serum chemistry profile. Vet Clin North Am Food Anim Pract 2007;23:403–26, v.
2. Goff J. Major advances in our understanding of nutritional influences on bovine health. J Dairy Sci 2006;89:1292–301.

3. Overton TR, McArt JAA, Nydam DV. A 100-Year Review: Metabolic health indicators and management of dairy cattle. J Dairy Sci 2017;100:10398–417.

4. LeBlanc S, Lissemore K, Kelton D, et al. Major advances in disease prevention in dairy cattle. J Dairy Sci 2006;89:1267–79.

5. Eckersall PD, Bell R. Acute phase proteins: Biomarkers of infection and inflammation in veterinary medicine. Vet J 2010;185:23–7.

6. Payne J, Dew SM, Manston R, et al. The use of a metabolic profile test in dairy herds. Vet Rec 1970;87:150–8.

7. Payne JM, Rowlands GJ, Manston R, et al. A Statistical Appraisal of the Results of Metabolic Profile Tests on 75 Dairy Herds. Br Vet J 1973;129:370–81.

8. Payne JM, Rowlands GJ, Manston R, et al. A Statistical Appraisal of the Results of the Metabolic Profile Tests on 191 Herds in the B.V.A./A.D.A.S Joint Exercise in Animal Health and Productivity. Br Vet J 1974;130:34–44.

9. Ferreira MFL, Renno LN, Rodrigues II, et al. Effects of parity order on performance, metabolic, and hormonal parameters of grazing beef cows during pre-calving and lactation periods. BMC Vet Res 2021;17:311.

10. Watanabe U, Takagi M, Yamato O, et al. Metabolic profile of Japanese black breeding cattle herds: usefulness in selection for nutrient supplementation to enhance reproductive performance and regional differences. J Vet Med Sci 2012;12:0441.

11. Celi P, Di Trana A, Claps S. Effects of perinatal nutrition on lactational performance, metabolic and hormonal profiles of dairy goats and respective kids. Small Ruminant Res 2008;79:129–36.

12. Ismail ZA, Al-Majali AM, Amireh F, et al. Metabolic profiles in goat does in late pregnancy with and without subclinical pregnancy toxemia. Vet Clin Pathol 2008;37:434–7.

13. Castillo C, Abuelo A, Hernández J. Usefulness of metabolic profiling in the assessment of the flock's health status and productive performance. Small Ruminant Res 2016;142:28–30.

14. N.D. Metabolic profiling. Segen's Medical Dictionary 2011. Available at: https://medical-dictionary.thefreedictionary.com/metabolic+profiling. Accessed July 11, 2022.

15. Rowlands G. A review of variations in the concentrations of metabolites in the blood of beef and dairy cattle associated with physiology, nutrition and disease, with particular reference to the interpretation of metabolic profiles. World Rev Nutr Diet 1980;35:172–235.

16. Herdt T, Dart B, Neuder L. Will large dairy herds lead to the revival of metabolic profile testing? In Am Assoc Bovine Pract Proc 34th Annu Conf 2001;27–34.

17. Shenkin A. Trace elements and inflammatory response: implications for nutritional support. Nutrition (Burbank, Los Angeles County, Calif) 1995;11:100–5.

18. Bradford B. Inflammation and transition cow disorders. Four-State Dairy Nutr Management Conf 2009;76:76–81.

19. Van Saun RJ, Wustenberg M. Metabolic profiling to evaluate nutritional and disease status. Bovine Pract 1997;31(2):37–42.

20. Oetzel GR. Undertaking nutritional diagnostic investigations. Vet Clin North Am Food Anim Pract 2014;30:765–88.

21. Smith RF, Oultram J, Dobson H. Herd monitoring to optimise fertility in the dairy cow: making the most of herd records, metabolic profiling and ultrasonography (research into practice). Animal 2014;8(Suppl 1):185–98.

22. Blowey R. Metabolic profiles–some aspects of their interpretation and use in the field. Vet Annu 1973.

23. Blowey R. A practical application of metabolic profiles. Vet Rec 1975;97(17): 324–7.

24. Macrae A, Whitaker D, Burrough E, et al. Use of metabolic profiles for the assessment of dietary adequacy in UK dairy herds. Vet Rec 2006;159:655–61.

25. Šamanc H, Kirovski D, Stojić V, et al. Application of the metabolic profile test in the prediction and diagnosis of fatty liver in Holstein cows. Acta veterinaria 2011;61:543–53.

26. Kida K. The metabolic profile test: its practicability in assessing feeding management and periparturient diseases in high yielding commercial dairy herds. J Vet Med Sci 2002;64:557–63.

27. Adams R, Stout W, Kradel D, et al. Use and limitations of profiles in assessing health or nutritional status of dairy herds. J Dairy Sci 1978;61:1671–9.

28. Lee A, Twardock A, Bubar R, et al. Blood metabolic profiles: their use and relation to nutritional status of dairy cows. J Dairy Sci 1978;61:1652–70.

29. Jones G, Wildman E, Troutt H Jr, et al. Metabolic profiles in Virginia dairy herds of different milk yields. J Dairy Sci 1982;65:683–8.

30. Gross JJ. Limiting factors for milk production in dairy cows: perspectives from physiology and nutrition. J Anim Sci 2022;100:1–11.

31. Horst EA, Kvidera SK, Baumgard LH. Invited review: The influence of immune activation on transition cow health and performance-A critical evaluation of traditional dogmas. J Dairy Sci 2021;104:8380–410.

32. Bell AW. Regulation of organic nutrient metabolism during transition from late pregnancy to early lactation. J Anim Sci 1995;73:2804–19.

33. Drackley JK, Dann HM, Douglas N, et al. Physiological and pathological adaptations in dairy cows that may increase susceptibility to periparturient diseases and disorders. Ital J Anim Sci 2005;4:323–44.

34. Mezzetti M, Cattaneo L, Passamonti MM, et al. The Transition Period Updated: A Review of the New Insights into the Adaptation of Dairy Cows to the New Lactation. Dairy 2021;2:617–36.

35. Chapinal N, Carson M, Duffield TF, et al. The association of serum metabolites with clinical disease during the transition period. J Dairy Sci 2011;94:4897–903.

36. Gross JJ, Kessler EC, Albrecht C, et al. Response of the cholesterol metabolism to a negative energy balance in dairy cows depends on the lactational stage. PLoS One 2015;10:e0121956.

37. Hussein HA, Thurmann JP, Staufenbiel R. 24-h variations of blood serum metabolites in high yielding dairy cows and calves. BMC Vet Res 2020;16:327.

38. Law RA, Young FJ, Patterson DC, et al. Effect of precalving and postcalving dietary energy level on performance and blood metabolite concentrations of dairy cows throughout lactation. J Dairy Sci 2011;94:808–23.

39. McArt JA, Nydam DV, Oetzel GR, et al. Elevated non-esterified fatty acids and beta-hydroxybutyrate and their association with transition dairy cow performance. Vet J 2013;198:560–70.

40. Tian H, Wang W, Zheng N, et al. Identification of diagnostic biomarkers and metabolic pathway shifts of heat-stressed lactating dairy cows. J Proteomics 2015;125:17–28.

41. Kida K. Relationships of metabolic profiles to milk production and feeding in dairy cows. J Vet Med Sci 2003;65:671–7.

42. Krogh MA, Hostens M, Salavati M, et al. Between- and within-herd variation in blood and milk biomarkers in Holstein cows in early lactation. Animal 2020;14: 1067–75.

43. Walter LL, Gartner T, Gernand E, et al. Effects of Parity and Stage of Lactation on Trend and Variability of Metabolic Markers in Dairy Cows. Animals (Basel) 2022; 12(8):1008.

44. Stokol T, Nydam DV. Effect of Anticoagulant and Storage Conditions on Bovine Nonesterified Fatty Acid and β-Hydroxybutyrate Concentrations in Blood. J Dairy Sci 2005;88:3139–44.

45. Leroy JL, Bossaert P, Opsomer G, et al. The effect of animal handling procedures on the blood non-esterified fatty acid and glucose concentrations of lactating dairy cows. Vet J 2011;187:81–4.

46. Herdt TH. Variability characteristics and test selection in herdlevel nutritional and metabolic profile testing. Vet Clin North America: Food Anim Pract 2000; 16:387–403.

47. Goff J, Horst R. Physiological changes at parturition and their relationship to metabolic disorders. J Dairy Sci 1997;80:1260–8.

48. Bauman DE, Currie WB. Partitioning of nutrients during pregnancy and lactation: a review of mechanisms involving homeostasis and homeorhesis. J Dairy Sci 1980;63:1514–29.

49. Reinhardt TA, Lippolis JD, McCluskey BJ, et al. Prevalence of subclinical hypocalcemia in dairy herds. Vet J 2011;188:122–4.

50. Andersson L. Subclinical ketosis in dairy cows. Vet Clin north america: Food Anim Pract 1988;4:233–51.

51. Van Saun RJ. Indicators of dairy cow transition risks: Metabolic profiling revisited. Tierarztl Prax Ausg G Grosstiere Nutztiere 2016;44:118–26, quiz 127.

52. Ospina PA, Nydam DV, Stokol T, et al. Evaluation of nonesterified fatty acids and beta-hydroxybutyrate in transition dairy cattle in the northeastern United States: Critical thresholds for prediction of clinical diseases. J Dairy Sci 2010;93: 546–54.

53. Barletta RV, Maturana Filho M, Carvalho PD, et al. Association of changes among body condition score during the transition period with NEFA and BHBA concentrations, milk production, fertility, and health of Holstein cows. Theriogenology 2017;104:30–6.

54. Geishauser T, Leslie K, Duffield T, et al. The association between selected metabolic parameters and left abomasal displacement in dairy cows. J Vet Med Ser A 1998;45:499–511.

55. Zarrin M, Grossen-Rosti L, Bruckmaier RM, et al. Elevation of blood beta-hydroxybutyrate concentration affects glucose metabolism in dairy cows before and after parturition. J Dairy Sci 2017;100:2323–33.

56. van der Drift SGA, Houweling M, Schonewille JT, et al. Protein and fat mobilization and associations with serum beta-hydroxybutyrate concentrations in dairy cows. J Dairy Sci 2012;95:4911–20.

57. McCarthy MM, Mann S, Nydam DV, et al. Short communication: concentrations of nonesterified fatty acids and beta-hydroxybutyrate in dairy cows are not well correlated during the transition period. J Dairy Sci 2015;98:6284–90.

58. Hoff B, Duffield T. Nutritional and metabolic profile testing of dairy cows. AHL LabNote 2015; Number 4. Available at: https://www.uoguelph.ca/ahl/ahl-labnote-4-nutritional-and-metabolic-profile-testing-dairy-cows. Accessed July 5, 2022.

59. Melendez P, Marin MP, Robles J, et al. Relationship between serum nonesterified fatty acids at calving and the incidence of periparturient diseases in Holstein dairy cows. Theriogenology 2009;72:826–33.

60. Hayirli A. The role of exogenous insulin in the complex of hepatic lipidosis and ketosis associated with insulin resistance phenomenon in postpartum dairy cattle. Vet Res Commun 2006;30:749–74.

61. De Koster JD, Opsomer G. Insulin resistance in dairy cows. Vet Clin North Am Food Anim Pract 2013;29:299–322.

62. Duffield T. Subclinical Ketosis in Lactating Dairy Cattle. Vet Clin North America: Food Anim Pract 2000;16:231–53.

63. Foster L. Clinical ketosis. Vet Clin North America: Food Anim Pract 1988;4: 253–67.

64. Mansion R, Rowlands GJ, Little W, et al. Variability of the blood composition of dairy cows in relation to time of day. J Agric Sci 2009;96:593–8.

65. Tatone EH, Gordon JL, Hubbs J, et al. A systematic review and meta-analysis of the diagnostic accuracy of point-of-care tests for the detection of hyperketonemia in dairy cows. Prev Vet Med 2016;130:18–32.

66. Benedet A, Manuelian CL, Zidi A, et al. Invited review: beta-hydroxybutyrate concentration in blood and milk and its associations with cow performance. Animal 2019;13:1676–89.

67. Piccione G, Messina V, Schembari A, et al. Pattern of serum protein fractions in dairy cows during different stages of gestation and lactation. J Dairy Res 2011; 78:421–5.

68. Alberghina D, Giannetto C, Vazzana I, et al. Reference intervals for total protein concentration, serum protein fractions, and albumin/globulin ratios in clinically healthy dairy cows. J Vet Diagn Invest 2011;23:111–4.

69. Cattaneo L, Lopreiato V, Piccioli-Cappelli F, et al. Plasma albumin-to-globulin ratio before dry-off as a possible index of inflammatory status and performance in the subsequent lactation in dairy cows. J Dairy Sci 2021;104:8228–42.

70. Bertoni G, Trevisi E, Han X, et al. Effects of inflammatory conditions on liver activity in puerperium period and consequences for performance in dairy cows. J Dairy Sci 2008;91:3300–10.

71. Bionaz M, Trevisi E, Calamari L, et al. Plasma paraoxonase, health, inflammatory conditions, and liver function in transition dairy cows. J Dairy Sci 2007;90: 1740–50.

72. Bertoni G, Trevisi E. Use of the liver activity index and other metabolic variables in the assessment of metabolic health in dairy herds. Vet Clin North Am Food Anim Pract 2013;29:413–31.

73. Bobe G, Young J, Beitz D. Invited review: pathology, etiology, prevention, and treatment of fatty liver in dairy cows. J Dairy Sci 2004;87:3105–24.

74. Holtenius P, Hjort M. Studies on the pathogenesis of fatty liver in cows. Bovine Pract 1990;25:91–4.

75. DeGaris PJ, Lean IJ. Milk fever in dairy cows: a review of pathophysiology and control principles. Vet J 2008;176:58–69.

76. Goff JP. The monitoring, prevention, and treatment of milk fever and subclinical hypocalcemia in dairy cows. Vet J 2008;176:50–7.

77. Lean IJ, Santos JEP, Block E, et al. Effects of prepartum dietary cation-anion difference intake on production and health of dairy cows: A meta-analysis. J Dairy Sci 2019;102:2103–33.

78. Lean IJ, Saun RV, Degaris PJ. Mineral and antioxidant management of transition dairy cows. Vet Clin North Am Food Anim Pract 2013;29:367–86.

79. Wilkens MR, Nelson CD, Hernandez LL, et al. Symposium review: Transition cow calcium homeostasis-Health effects of hypocalcemia and strategies for prevention. J Dairy Sci 2020;103:2909–27.

80. Curtis C, Erb H, Sniffen C, et al. Association of parturient hypocalcemia with eight periparturient disorders in Holstein cows. J Am Vet Assoc 1983;183: 559–61.

81. Martinez N, Sinedino LD, Bisinotto RS, et al. Effect of induced subclinical hypocalcemia on physiological responses and neutrophil function in dairy cows. J Dairy Sci 2014;97:874–87.

82. Rodriguez EM, Aris A, Bach A. Associations between subclinical hypocalcemia and postparturient diseases in dairy cows. J Dairy Sci 2017;100:7427–34.

83. Valldecabres A, Silva-Del-Rio N. Association of low serum calcium concentration after calving with productive and reproductive performance in multiparous Jersey cows. J Dairy Sci 2021;104:11983–94.

84. Venjakob PL, Staufenbiel R, Heuwieser W, et al. Association between serum calcium dynamics around parturition and common postpartum diseases in dairy cows. J Dairy Sci 2021;104:2243–53.

85. Grunberg W. Treatment of phosphorus balance disorders. Vet Clin North Am Food Anim Pract 2014;30:383–408, vi.

86. Grunberg W, Scherpenisse P, Cohrs I, et al. Phosphorus content of muscle tissue and muscle function in dairy cows fed a phosphorus-deficient diet during the transition period. J Dairy Sci 2019;102:4072–93.

87. Ordway R, Ishler V, Varga G. Effects of sucrose supplementation on dry matter intake, milk yield, and blood metabolites of periparturient Holstein dairy cows. J Dairy Sci 2002;85:879–88.

88. Vallimont J, Varga G, Arieli A, et al. Effects of prepartum somatotropin and monensin on metabolism and production of periparturient Holstein dairy cows. J Dairy Sci 2001;84:2607–21.

89. Van Saun R, Todd A, Varga G. Serum mineral concentrations and risk of periparturient disease. In Am Assoc Bovine Pract Proc 38th Annu Conf 2005;178–9.

90. Van Saun RJ, Todd A, Varga G. Serum mineral concentrations and periparturient disease in Holstein dairy cows. Prod Dis 2006;221.

91. Herdt TH, Hoff B. The use of blood analysis to evaluate trace mineral status in ruminant livestock. Vet Clin North Am Food Anim Pract 2011;27:255–83, vii.

92. Goff JP, Kimura K, Horst RL. Effect of mastectomy on milk fever, energy, and vitamins A, E, and β-carotene status at parturition. J Dairy Sci 2002;85:1427–36.

93. Weiss W, Hogan J, Todhunter D, et al. Effect of vitamin E supplementation in diets with a low concentration of selenium on mammary gland health of dairy cows. J Dairy Sci 1997;80:1728–37.

94. LeBlanc S, Herdt T, Seymour W, et al. Peripartum serum vitamin E, retinol, and beta-carotene in dairy cattle and their associations with disease. J Dairy Sci 2004;87:609–19.

95. Omur A, Kirbas A, Aksu E, et al. Effects of antioxidant vitamins (A, D, E) and trace elements (Cu, Mn, Se, Zn) on some metabolic and reproductive profiles in dairy cows during transition period. Polish J Vet Sci 2016;19:697–706.

96. Sayiner S, Darbaz I, Ergene O, et al. Changes in antioxidant enzyme activities and metabolic parameters in dairy cows during different reproductive periods. Theriogenology 2021;159:116–22.

97. Mutinati M, Piccinno M, Roncetti M, et al. Oxidative stress during pregnancy in the sheep. Reprod Domest Anim 2013;48:353–7.

98. Bradford BJ, Swartz TH. Review: Following the smoke signals: inflammatory signaling in metabolic homeostasis and homeorhesis in dairy cattle. Animal 2020;14:s144–54.

99. Bradford BJ, Yuan K, Farney JK, et al. Invited review: Inflammation during the transition to lactation: New adventures with an old flame. J Dairy Sci 2015;98: 6631–50.

100. Sordillo LM, Raphael W. Significance of metabolic stress, lipid mobilization, and inflammation on transition cow disorders. Vet Clin North Am Food Anim Pract 2013;29:267–78.

101. Huzzey JM, Duffield TF, LeBlanc SJ, et al. Short communication: Haptoglobin as an early indicator of metritis. J Dairy Sci 2009;92:621–5.

102. Nightingale CR, Sellers MD, Ballou MA. Elevated plasma haptoglobin concentrations following parturition are associated with elevated leukocyte responses and decreased subsequent reproductive efficiency in multiparous Holstein dairy cows. Vet Immunol Immunopathol 2015;164:16–23.

103. Bannikov GA, Hinds CA, Rajala-Schultz PJ, et al. Serum haptoglobin-matrix metalloproteinase 9 (Hp-MMP 9) complex as a biomarker of systemic inflammation in cattle. Vet Immunol Immunopathol 2011;139:41–9.

104. Schmitt R, Pieper L, Gonzalez-Grajales LA, et al. Evaluation of different acute-phase proteins for herd health diagnostics in early postpartum Holstein Friesian dairy cows. J Dairy Res 2021;88:33–7.

105. Trevisi E, Amadori M, Cogrossi S, et al. Metabolic stress and inflammatory response in high-yielding, periparturient dairy cows. Res Vet Sci 2012;93: 695–704.

106. Maas J. Diagnostic considerations for evaluating nutritional problems in cattle. Vet Clin North Am Food Anim Pract 2007;23:527–39, vi-vii.

107. Cozzi G, Ravarotto L, Gottardo F, et al. Short communication: reference values for blood parameters in Holstein dairy cows: effects of parity, stage of lactation, and season of production. J Dairy Sci 2011;94:3895–901.

108. Piccione G, Messina V, Marafioti S, et al. Changes of some haematochemical parameters in dairy cows during late gestation, post partum, lactation and dry periods. Vet Med Zoot 2012;58:59–64.

109. Brscic M, Cozzi G, Lora I, et al. Short communication: Reference limits for blood analytes in Holstein late-pregnant heifers and dry cows: Effects of parity, days relative to calving, and season. J Dairy Sci 2015;98:7886–92.

110. Mann S, McArt J. Abuelo Ã. Metabolic disease testing on farms: epidemiological principles. In Pract 2020;42:405–14.

111. Chapinal N, Leblanc SJ, Carson ME, et al. Herd-level association of serum metabolites in the transition period with disease, milk production, and early lactation reproductive performance. J Dairy Sci 2012;95:5676–82.

112. Oetzel GR. Monitoring and testing dairy herds for metabolic disease. Vet Clin North Am Food Anim Pract 2004;20:651–74.

113. Ospina PA, Nydam DV, Stokol T, et al. Association between the proportion of sampled transition cows with increased nonesterified fatty acids and beta-hydroxybutyrate and disease incidence, pregnancy rate, and milk production at the herd level. J Dairy Sci 2010;93:3595–601.

114. Duffield T, LeBlanc S. Interpretation of serum metabolic parameters around the transition period. Southwest Nutrition and Management Conference, February 26, 2009, 106–114, Chandler, AZ.

115. Ospina PA, McArt JA, Overton TR, et al. Using nonesterified fatty acids and beta-hydroxybutyrate concentrations during the transition period for herd-level monitoring of increased risk of disease and decreased reproductive and milking performance. Vet Clin North Am Food Anim Pract 2013;29:387–412.

116. Kronfeld D, Donoghue S, Copp R, et al. Nutritional status of dairy cows indicated by analysis of blood. J Dairy Sci 1982;65:1925–33.

117. Van Saun RJ. Use and interpretation of pooled metabolic profiles for evaluating transition cow health status. In Am Assoc Bovine Pract Proc 38th Annu Conf 2005;180:180.

118. Borchardt S, Staufenbiel R. Evaluation of the use of nonesterified fatty acids and β-hydroxybutyrate concentrations in pooled serum samples for herd-based detection of subclinical ketosis in dairy cows during the first week after parturition. J Am Vet Med Assoc 2012;240:1003–11.

119. Hussein HA, Westphal A, Staufenbiel R. Pooled serum sample metabolic profiling as a screening tool in dairy herds with a history of ketosis or milk fever. Comp Clin Pathol 2012;22:1075–82.

120. Humann-Ziehank E, Tegtmeyer PC, Seelig B, et al. Variation of serum selenium concentrations in German sheep flocks and implications for herd health management consultancy. Acta Veterinaria Scand 2013;55:1–8.

121. Lehwenich T. Investigation to the use of metabolic profile test in herd management of dairy cattle. Berlin, FU: Veterinärmed Fak; 1999.

122. De Vries A, Reneau J. Application of statistical process control charts to monitor changes in animal production systems. J Anim Sci 2010;88:E11–24.

123. Ingraham RH. L.C. K. Metabolic profiling. Vet Clin North Am Food Anim Pract 1988;4:391–411.

124. De Koster J, Salavati M, Grelet C, et al. Prediction of metabolic clusters in early-lactation dairy cows using models based on milk biomarkers. J Dairy Sci 2019; 102:2631–44.

125. Gross JJ, Bruckmaier RM. Review: Metabolic challenges in lactating dairy cows and their assessment via established and novel indicators in milk. Animal 2019; 13:s75–81.

126. Fukumori R, Taguchi T, Oetzel GR, et al. Performance evaluation of a newly designed on-farm blood testing system for determining blood non-esterified fatty acid and beta-hydroxybutyrate concentrations in dairy cows. Res Vet Sci 2021;135:247–52.

127. Luke TDW, Rochfort S, Wales WJ, et al. Metabolic profiling of early-lactation dairy cows using milk mid-infrared spectra. J Dairy Sci 2019;102:1747–60.

128. Calamari L, Ferrari A, Minuti A, et al. Assessment of the main plasma parameters included in a metabolic profile of dairy cow based on Fourier Transform mid-infrared spectroscopy: preliminary results. BMC Vet Res 2016;12:4.

129. Sun LW, Zhang HY, Wu L, et al. (1)H-Nuclear magnetic resonance-based plasma metabolic profiling of dairy cows with clinical and subclinical ketosis. J Dairy Sci 2014;97:1552–62.

130. Giannuzzi D, Mota LFM, Pegolo S, et al. In-line near-infrared analysis of milk coupled with machine learning methods for the daily prediction of blood metabolic profile in dairy cattle. Sci Rep 2022;12:8058.

131. Mantysaari P, Juga J, Lidauer MH, et al. The relationships between early lactation energy status indicators and endocrine fertility traits in dairy cows. J Dairy Sci 2022;105(8):6833–44. https://doi.org/10.3168/jds.2021-21077.

132. Abuelo A, Hernandez J, Benedito JL, et al. Oxidative stress index (OSi) as a new tool to assess redox status in dairy cattle during the transition period. Animal 2013;7:1374–8.

133. Hailemariam D, Mandal R, Saleem F, et al. Identification of predictive biomarkers of disease state in transition dairy cows. J Dairy Sci 2014;97:2680–93.

134. Putman AK, Brown JL, Gandy JC, et al. Changes in biomarkers of nutrient metabolism, inflammation, and oxidative stress in dairy cows during the transition into the early dry period. J Dairy Sci 2018;101:9350–9.
135. Rico JE, Bandaru VV, Dorskind JM, et al. Plasma ceramides are elevated in overweight Holstein dairy cows experiencing greater lipolysis and insulin resistance during the transition from late pregnancy to early lactation. J Dairy Sci 2015;98:7757–70.
136. Wang Y, Gao Y, Xia C, et al. Pathway analysis of plasma different metabolites for dairy cow ketosis. Ital J Anim Sci 2016;15:545–51.
137. Ishikawa S, Ikuta K, Obara Y, et al. Cluster analysis to evaluate disease risk in periparturient dairy cattle. Anim Sci J 2020;91:e13442.
138. Ceciliani F, Lecchi C, Urh C, et al. Proteomics and metabolomics characterizing the pathophysiology of adaptive reactions to the metabolic challenges during the transition from late pregnancy to early lactation in dairy cows. J Proteomics 2018;178:92–106.
139. Luo ZZ, Shen LH, Jiang J, et al. Plasma metabolite changes in dairy cows during parturition identified using untargeted metabolomics. J Dairy Sci 2019;102:4639–50.
140. Ghaffari MH, Jahanbekam A, Sadri H, et al. Metabolomics meets machine learning: Longitudinal metabolite profiling in serum of normal versus overconditioned cows and pathway analysis. J Dairy Sci 2019;102:11561–85.
141. Ghaffari MH, Schuh K, Kules J, et al. Plasma proteomic profiling and pathway analysis of normal and overconditioned dairy cows during the transition from late pregnancy to early lactation. J Dairy Sci 2020;103:4806–21.

The Role of Histopathology in Ruminant Diagnostics

Matthew M. Hille, DVM, PhD*, Sarah J. Sillman, DVM, PhD, Dip. ACVP,
Bruce W. Brodersen, DVM, PhD

KEYWORDS

- Histopathology • Ruminants • Diagnostic pathology • Abortion • Enteric
- Bovine respiratory disease

KEY POINTS

- Some diseases *require* histopathology for a definitive diagnosis.
- A methodical approach to tissue sampling improves the success of histopathology diagnoses.
- When available, a detailed clinical history is crucial to assigning significance to subtle histologic lesions.

INTRODUCTION

Despite advancements in veterinary diagnostic techniques, particularly in molecular biology, veterinary pathologists still spend a large part of their time performing histologic examinations of tissues to investigate animal disease. Even in ruminants, where the focus of disease investigation is most often on promoting overall herd health and less focused on individual animal health, histopathology can provide a wealth of information that can be crucial to the diagnostician in obtaining a definitive diagnosis. When used with other available diagnostic testing methods, histopathology can provide definitive (eg, visualization of an agent), confirmatory (eg, evidence of bronchopneumonia in a lung that was polymerase chain reaction (PCR) positive for a known respiratory pathogen), or supplemental information (eg, degree of chronicity). Despite the rapid advancement and sensitivity of tests that rely on nucleic acid detection, as well as the construction of multiplex assays that probe for numerous agents at one time, histopathology remains an important method to confirm or rule out detected agents as a likely cause of disease. This is especially important in ruminant diseases where many times we are dealing with opportunistic pathogens that can be detected

Nebraska Veterinary Diagnostic Center, School of Veterinary Medicine and Biomedical Sciences, University of Nebraska-Lincoln, 4040 East Campus Loop North, 115N NVDC, Lincoln, NE 68583-0907, USA
* Corresponding author.
E-mail address: mhille@unl.edu

Vet Clin Food Anim 39 (2023) 73–91
https://doi.org/10.1016/j.cvfa.2022.10.005
0749-0720/23/© 2022 Elsevier Inc. All rights reserved.

even in healthy animals. There are also disease processes such as polioencephaloma-lacia (PEM), bovine interstitial lung disease (BILD), and attaching and effacing *Escherichia coli,* which are examples of disease processes that, by definition, require histopathology to make a definitive diagnosis.

Histopathological Diagnosis and Sampling

An efficient histopathologic examination ideally relies on an adequate history of the health of the herd and individual animal, antemortem clinical signs, postmortem lesions, and proper tissue sampling, handling, and fixation. Effort should be made to maximize each of these components when possible. Purposefully omitting important information concerning the clinical history when submitting a diagnostic case (for any species) so as to not "bias the pathologist," helps no one, particularly the producer or owner, as clinical information and context can be critically important to developing a diagnosis. The one thing that is crucial to a histopathologic examination, however, is submitting the proper tissue(s). It is not uncommon for an incorrect clinical diagnosis to lead to only focused tissues being submitted, only to find out the clinical diagnosis was incorrect and the diagnostician is left with no other tissue to facilitate further investigation for the case.

Specific tissues to sample for organ systems are described in more detail below under specific organ system diseases, but it is good practice to have a routine set of tissues to obtain from every necropsy. In general, this should include heart, lung, liver, kidney, spleen, abomasum, rumen, intestine, and a lymph node. Other tissues should be added depending on the clinical history (ie, brain or spinal cord from a neurologic animal). Organ systems with no apparent gross lesions can be sampled randomly. When a gross lesion is observed, it is ideal to sample areas that include the suspected lesion, normal tissue, and the junction of normal to abnormal. **Fig. 1** indicates the suggested sampling sites following this principle. Proper tissue handling can be important to minimize artifacts within the tissue. This is particularly true for crush artifacts of lung and gastrointestinal tissue. Pressure applied to lung before fixation can induce artificial collapse of the lung alveoli which can mask lesions, or be misinterpreted as atelectasis. Trimming only undisturbed tissue directly into fixative, and discarding any

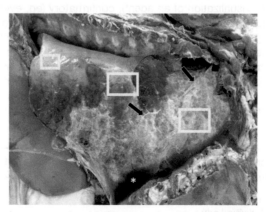

Fig. 1. Severe bronchopneumonia with fibrinous pleuritis and reducible adhesions (*arrows*) and pleural effusion (*asterisk*) in a feeder calf. Yellow boxes indicate the examples of tissue to sample to allow for both abnormal and normal tissue parenchyma to be examined histologically. (*Courtesy of* Scott Fritz.)

portion that was manipulated can help minimize the chances of a crush artifact being included in the tissue sample.

Tissue Fixation

A 10% formalin solution (1 part 37% formaldehyde: 9 parts water) is the fixative used by most of the practitioners when submitting histopathology samples. This solution can be either purchased commercially as a ready-to-use formulation, or made in the clinic. Although commercial formulations will be more uniform in terms of buffers and pH, do-it-yourself formulations can be more cost-effective, yet still provide adequate fixation assuming the proper ratios are used; 10% formalin penetrates bovine tissues at a rate of approximately 1 mm per hour.[1] Given this slow rate of penetration, tissue sample size is important to assure proper fixation. As a general rule, trying to limit tissue thickness to 10 mm (roughly the diameter of a pea) and having at least a 10:1 formalin to tissue volume ratio will yield adequate fixation that minimizes postmortem autolytic changes, particularly within the interior of the tissue. Most diagnosticians or veterinarians will obtain gastrointestinal samples last in a necropsy, to avoid cross-contamination of other tissues with intestinal contents. However, given the tendency for intestine to autolyze quickly, it may be indicated to obtain these samples first in cases where enteric disease is the most important concern in an effort to minimize autolysis. Ensuring immediate contact of the mucosal surface of intestine with formalin will also help to minimize autolysis. If tissue in formalin is allowed to freeze, this can cause substantial freeze artifact because of the buildup of ice crystals that induce cells to rupture, thus greatly disrupting their microscopic morphology. The addition of an alcohol such as ethanol, methanol, or isopropyl alcohol (1 part alcohol: 9 parts formalin) to formalin during winter months can help decrease the chances of freezing during transport without negatively affecting the fixation process. Regardless of environmental temperatures, shipping specimens in an insulated cooler is recommended to maintain temperature control.

Histopathological Nomenclature

An important component to the clinical interpretation of a histopathology report is to understand the categorization criteria for degrees of chronicity in inflammatory, degenerative, or reactive processes that are used in anatomic pathology. These terms do not always align exactly with how they are used clinically, and thus, may not agree with common usage in the field or veterinary clinic. For example, a calf with bovine respiratory disease (BRD) may manifest with clinical signs and die within a matter of hours, but lung tissue may have histologic evidence of a more chronic disease that went undetected. Understanding these differences can be crucial in determining vaccine or treatment failure or whether farm staff are simply missing sick calves. Some of the more clinically applicable criteria are briefly summarized here, and the reader is referred to other texts for a more detailed explanation of acute versus chronic inflammation at the microscopic level.[2,3] One of the main criteria in categorizing inflammatory lesions histologically is the relative abundance of the different inflammatory cells. Acute lesions involve mainly neutrophils as they are the first to respond to chemotactic influence, whereas mononuclear cells take longer to proliferate and respond and are therefore associated more so with chronic disease. The degree of fibrosis is another important histologic pattern with acute lesions having no to minimal amount of fibrosis, whereas chronic changes are often accompanied by appreciable fibrosis. The reason for this difference is that activated fibroblasts simply take time to lay down collagen, and therefore, the presence of collagen indicates a longer time since the initial tissue or cellular insult. As a general rule, acute implies an insult that is minutes or hours old (up to about 24–36 hours), whereas chronic implies a lesion that is days old or more. Although many of these characteristics seem to be objective, there is substantial subjectivity built into histologic interpretation because these characteristics are not absolute, but instead take place on a spectrum. For example, a lesion containing a majority of neutrophils, yet also a substantial amount of mononuclear cells along with mild fibrosis may represent the transition from acute to chronic. The term subacute is used to indicate that the lesion has characteristics of both acute and chronic lesions and most likely represents a snapshot in the transformation toward a chronic process.

THE APPLICATION OF HISTOPATHOLOGY IN SPECIFIC RUMINANT DISEASES

The remainder of this article discusses diseases of specific organ systems and highlights ruminant diseases where histopathology can be particularly valuable, with an emphasis on bovine diseases. Where applicable, histopathology submission or interpretation tips specific to the respective diseases will be highlighted. This article is not meant to be all inconclusive, and the reader is encouraged to communicate with their own diagnostic laboratory regarding preferred sampling and/or handling of tissues in unique cases.

Respiratory Disease

Perhaps the most important role histopathology plays in BRD investigations is the ability confirm or rule out the presence of lung disease. A thorough histologic examination of lung tissue involves assessing the morphology of the alveolar and airway epithelium, interstitium, vasculature, and pleura. Changes in one or a combination of these can help confirm lung disease and rule in or out certain etiologies. A prime example of this is in cases with evidence of vasculitis and interstitial inflammation without substantial airway involvement. These histologic characteristics are often seen in young calves with septicemia as a result of Salmonella spp or other gram-negative infection (Fig. 2) and can give the false clinical impression of primary lung disease as these calves are usually lethargic, febrile, and dyspneic. Determining septicemia versus bronchopneumonia is important for treatment and prevention strategies. Lungs can also seem consolidated and reddened grossly, only to find the lung parenchyma is within normal limits histologically. In these types of cases, there may be substantial congestion of the vasculature, giving the false gross appearance of overt lung disease. Pulmonary edema is another histologic change that is nonspecific, but can still be helpful in the overall etiologic determination. Common causes of pulmonary edema in ruminants include cardiac insufficiency, BRD, sepsis among others.[4–6] However, pulmonary edema is also a common finding in lung tissue with advanced postmortem autolysis, highlighting the importance of evaluating all tissue components grossly and histologically before deciding the relative significance of an individual lesion characteristic such as pulmonary edema. If pulmonary edema is suspected clinically, submission of heart and liver in addition to the lung will help determine the significance.

Advancements in testing based on the detection of pathogen nucleic acid in tissue specimens have greatly benefited BRD research and diagnostics. Testing for individual BRD pathogens by PCR has been available for some time, and more recently, multiplex assays have been developed to detect both viral and bacterial pathogens known to be associated with clinical BRD.[7,8] Being able to estimate the relative nucleic acid load of these pathogens in lung samples via cycle threshold (Ct) values is an extremely valuable tool for BRD diagnostic investigations. However, the presence of nucleic acid does not always confirm etiology. Histopathology is able to supplement

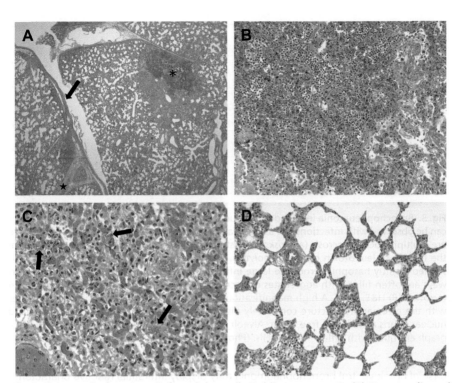

Fig. 2. Pneumonia due to sepsis from Salmonella Dublin serogroup D. (*A*) Hematoxylin and eosin (H&E), 12.5X. At low magnification, the alveoli and interstitium are expanded by inflammatory cells and edema. There are foci of more severe cellular influx mixed with large amounts of fibrin, neutrophils, and hemorrhage (*asterisk*). The pleural surface of an adjacent section of lung is moderately thickened (*arrow*), and there is moderate interlobular edema (*star*). (*B*) H&E, 200X. Higher magnification displaying a marked influx of leukocytes mixed with fibrin and hemorrhage. The hemosiderin within macrophages indicates previous hemorrhage and hemophagocytosis. (*C*) H&E, 400X. Numerous intravascular and extravascular aggregates of rod bacteria are present throughout the sections (*arrows*). (*D*) H&E, 200X. Areas much less affected from the same animal. The interstitium is moderately expanded by inflammatory cells and fibrin but there is minimal hemorrhage and/or necrosis. Areas like this example are evidence for the need to examine more than a single area in a diseased lung. (Photomicrographs courtesy of Matthew M. Hille.)

the data from these molecular diagnostic techniques and help determine whether a particular pathogen is likely to be involved. For example, the repeats-in-toxin that is secreted by *Mannheimia haemolytica* results in fairly consistent cytopathic effects that can be identified on microscopic examination of lung (**Fig. 3**). Seeing such lesions in a case with ancillary PCR testing that shows a high nucleic acid level for *M haemolytica* would suggest it is a primary pathogen involved in the case. Viral pathogens tend to predominantly affect the alveolar interstitium, whereas bacterial pathogens mostly affect the airway lumina, which results in either interstitial pneumonia or bronchopneumonia, respectively. It is extremely common to have mixed viral and bacterial infections in BRD cases, and bronchointerstitial pneumonia is the morphological diagnosis used when the interstitium and airways are both affected. An example of bronchointerstitial pneumonia due to primary infection with bovine respiratory syncytial virus (BRSV) is shown in **Fig. 4**. Furthermore, the caudodorsal portion of lungs in a

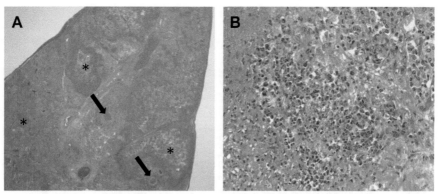

Fig. 3. Bronchopneumonia in a feeder calf due to *M haemolytica*. Similar microscopic lesions can be observed with infections by *Pasteurella multocida* and *H somni*. (*A*) H&E, 12.5X. There are multiple foci of necrosis (*asterisks*) consistent with the cytopathic effect resulting from the release of leukotoxin by *M haemolytica*. The vast majority of the lung parenchyma is stained slightly basophilic from the large influx of inflammatory cells that fill alveoli. Airways are often filled with aggregates of necrotic debris mixed with neutrophils and fibrin (*arrows*). (*B*) H&E, 400X. A high magnification view of a focus of necrosis within the center with the alveolar architecture completely disrupted and replaced by necrotic cellular and nuclear debris mixed with free fibrin. Alveoli in the upper right portion of the photomicrograph are filled with inflammatory cells. (Photomicrographs courtesy of Matthew M. Hille.)

case of cranioventral bronchopneumonia may display interstitial reactive characteristics, which highlights the importance of taking samples from different areas relative to gross lesions as described above. If the diagnostician is only able to examine sections of caudodorsal lung in such a case, they could be misled to incorrectly favor interstitial pneumonia as the primary diagnosis.

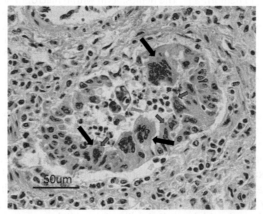

Fig. 4. Bronchointerstitial pneumonia in a feeder calf. There are syncytia (*black arrows*) and suspect eosinophilic cytoplasmic viral inclusion bodies (*red arrows*) within epithelial cells suggestive of bovine respiratory syncytial virus (BRSV). PCR testing on lung tissue resulted in Ct values of 15.88 for BRSV and 26.23 for bovine coronavirus (BoCV) indicating an exceptionally high level of BRSV within the sample. (Photomicrograph courtesy of Bruce W. Brodersen.)

The disease traditionally referred to as atypical interstitial pneumonia (AIP) requires histopathology, by definition, for a definitive diagnosis.[9] This disease, originally described formally more than 60 years ago,[10] has historically gone by a number of colloquial names including fog fever, dust pneumonia, and acute interstitial pneumonia among others. Recently, there has been an effort to change the nomenclature to "bovine interstitial lung disease" which the authors feel reflects the disease process more accurately. Pulmonary edema and congestion, emphysema, fibrosis, type II pneumocyte hyperplasia, and the presence of hyaline membranes lining the alveolar wall are the most frequent microscopic lesions observed.[11] Examples of gross and histopathological lesions associated with BILD are shown in **Fig. 5**. Suspected causes of BILD are numerous, and a recent VCNA publication provides an excellent review of this disease and potential causes.[9] There are no demonstrated treatments for BILD but the diagnosis is critical to (1) avoid unnecessary treatment to the rest of the herd or (2) determine whether a particular animal is a true representation of the herd-level disease. A diagnosis of interstitial lung disease in a feeder calf during a respiratory disease outbreak exhibiting severe morbidity and mortality would indicate additional diagnostics are warranted as BILD does not typically cause herd-level disease.

Cardiac Disease

When it comes to examination of the heart in ruminant disease investigations, histophilosis and toxic myocarditis are two of the most common disease processes encountered. Lymphoma commonly affects the heart in cattle, but does not pose the same time-sensitive risk to herdmates as does histophilosis or toxic myocarditis. Similarly, congestive heart failure has histologic characteristics that when coupled with clinical signs and gross lesions, can help confirm the diagnosis. If congestive heart failure is suspected, heart, lung, and liver should be submitted.

Myocardial inflammation, degeneration, and/or necrosis in ruminant cases of toxicosis can be caused by a number of different entities including via the ingestion of ionophores, gossypol, plants of the genus *Senna* such as coffee senna (*Senna occidentalis*), and Japanese yew (*Taxus cuspidate*) among others.[4,12–14] In the authors' experience, ionophore toxicosis, particularly from monensin, is the most commonly encountered cause of toxic myocardial disease in ruminants in the Great

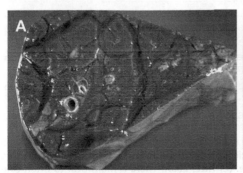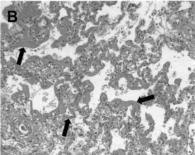

Fig. 5. Bovine interstitial lung disease (formerly AIP). (*A*) The disease can present with variable gross lesions, but heavy, wet lungs with pronounced interlobular edema are a common finding. Image credit: Noah's Arkive, F00841, submitted by Allison. (*B*) H&E, 20X. The interstitium is expanded by a moderate number of leukocytes. Alveoli are lined by variably thick hyaline membranes (*arrows*). (Photomicrograph courtesy of Matthew M. Hille.)

Plains. Although cattle are not as sensitive to ionophores as monogastrics, and they are widely used, cattle are susceptible to toxicosis when exposed to levels above those recommended in feed. Cases of ionophore toxicosis often involve either a mistake during formulation or human error in either mixing or when it is administered as a top dressing. Cases usually occur after a single exposure to a toxic dose and exhibit monophasic changes within the myocardium that helps to distinguish from etiologies that are characterized by polyphasic changes, which are more often the result of chronic, low-level exposure to an insult. Examples of gross and histologic lesions in

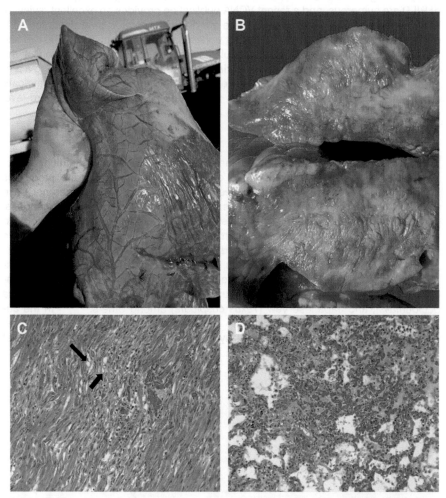

Fig. 6. Gross and histopathologic lesions from a case of numerous unexpected deaths in a pen of feeder cattle due to monensin toxicosis. (*A*) Severe pulmonary edema. (*B*) Coalescing areas of pale myocardium on cut surface. (*C*) H&E, 200X. There is multifocal to often coalescing myocardial necrosis with few leukocytes. Note the cytoplasmic vacuolation (*arrows*) and loss of appreciable striations within the necrotic and degenerating myocytes, whereas the nuclei remain relatively intact, indicative of a subacute process. (*D*) H&E, 200X. The lung is moderately congested. Alveoli are partially to completely fill with homogenous proteinaceous fluid (edema fluid). (Photos and photomicrographs courtesy of Matthew M. Hille.)

confirmed cases of monensin toxicosis of feeder cattle are shown in **Fig. 6**. The toxic effects of monensin in skeletal muscle is due to the disruption of the Na^+/K^+ ATPase and Ca^{2+} ATPase enzymatic function, which is the same mechanism of action in the apicomplexan parasites that are the intended target.[15] Therefore, cardiac muscle lesions are more frequently observed, presumably due to the comparatively increased workload and energy demand of the myocardium. In addition, within the heart, the papillary muscle is the best choice for tissue sampling for the same reason. Given the importance of histologic examination of heart muscle in cases of toxic myocardial disease, fixed samples of heart from all carcasses during an outbreak of unexpected deaths suspected to be due to ionophore toxicosis should be obtained.

Ruminants infected with *Histophilus somni* can manifest with a number of different disease processes including respiratory disease, pleuritis, polyarthritis, necrotizing myocarditis, thrombotic meningoencephalitis (TME), and as an opportunistic abortifacient pathogen causing reproductive losses.[16–19] Historically, histophilosis was regarded as a disease of cattle in Canada and the northern United States, but *H somni* is commonly isolated from bovine cases at the Nebraska Veterinary Diagnostic Center (NVDC) from a wide geographic area. In calendar year 2021, 31.58% of bovine multiplex PCR tests at the NVDC were positive for *H somni*. In addition, according to the most recent Academy of Veterinary Consultants diagnostic laboratory report for bovine cases submitted November 2018–April 2019, the PCR positive rate for *H somni* was substantial in diagnostic laboratories from Georgia (37.0%), Iowa (67.98%), and Texas (47.6%) which supports the fact that histophilosis is not just a disease of particularly cold climates.

The cardiac lesions associated with sudden death from histophilosis can be seen alone or in combination with lesions in the central nervous system, lungs, or joints. These lesions can range from small areas of myocardial degeneration and infarction, to large areas of abscessation that can be easily observed grossly (**Fig. 7**). Much like ionophore toxicosis, the papillary muscles of the heart are a key location of lesion development in histophilosis (**Fig. 8**). For this reason, it is always a good idea to make serial slices through a heart for visual inspection in a case of sudden death where histophilosis is suspected clinically. An area that is discolored (either darker or lighter than normal), or abscessed, is a prime sample for PCR and histologic analysis to help confirm the diagnosis.

Over time, there has been an apparent decrease in the incidence of TME and an increase in the incidence of sudden death due to the myocarditis form, particularly in feedlot animals.[16] The authors' clinical and diagnostic experience would support the notion that the myocarditis form is currently the most clinically important systemic form observed in cattle, whereas there has been, at least anecdotally, a decrease in the number of TME cases. This switch from the TME form to the myocarditis form of *H somni* infection may be due to pathogen genetics, however, a detailed understanding of the variation in *H somni* is lacking.[20] Enhanced understanding of *H somni* genomics may help to understand differences in disease types and enhance preventative strategies, such as vaccination.[21]

Neurologic Disease

The evaluation of neurologic disease in the bovine at postmortem examination is most rewarding when performed with a detailed clinical history and neurologic examination. Nervous system tissues are functionally and structurally complex, such that considerable effort and cost can be saved with antemortem neuroanatomic localization of lesions. The bovine brain and spinal cord are extensive and complex, and multifocal lesions can easily be missed if not scrutinized clinically along with a postmortem

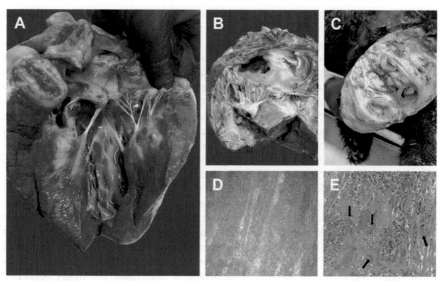

Fig. 7. Gross and histologic lesions consistent with the systemic form of *H somni* infection. (*A*) Papillary myocarditis and infarction. (*B*) Abscessation within the incised papillary muscle. (*C*) Severe, chronic suppurative arthritis in the same calf as (*A*). (*D*) H&E, 100X. Severe necrosuppurative myocarditis due to *H somni* from the same calf as 7A and 7C. There is a marked influx of neutrophils, macrophages and lymphocytes with myocardial necrosis and replacement. Intact myocytes are mostly hypereosinophilic and swollen. (*E*) H&E, 400X. Higher magnification photomicrograph showing the marked infiltration of inflammatory cells that often replaces the myocardium. There are innumerable aggregates of coccobacilli throughout the section (*arrows*). (Photos and photomicrographs: Photomicrograph Courtesy of Matthew M. Hille (7A, 7C, 7D, 7E), Courtesy of Scott Fritz (7B).)

survey of tissues. The clinician should always be mindful that metabolic or toxic etiologies of "nervous system signs" can be functional in origin and leave no anatomic nervous system lesion. Therefore, a thorough histopathology examination demonstrating no lesions still provides valuable content and can help verify the clinical suspect, for example, with botulism or tetanus.

One of the common problems encountered with histopathology of the brain and spinal cord is poorly directed or incomplete sampling. A brief tutorial on the removal of the

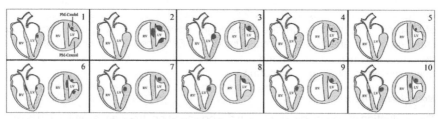

Fig. 8. An illustration of the anatomic location of 10 cases of cardiac histophilosis showing the tendency for lesion development within the left ventricular papillary muscle. A close gross examination of serial sections of the papillary muscles is a good approach if histophilosis is suspected. (Cartoon originally from O'toole, D., and Sondgeroth, K.S. (2016). Histophilosis as a Natural Disease. Curr Top Microbiol Immunol (396) 15-48. Used here with the author's (O'toole) permission.)

brain in the field using an axe is discussed elsewhere with pictures.[22] After removal from the skull, it is ideal to serially section the brain to evaluate the extent of the neuropil for malacia (softening), hemorrhage, abscesses, and other lesions. It is advantageous to inspect the ventral aspect of the brain for pituitary abscessation. Abnormal tissue, in addition to representative samples from cerebral cortex, cerebellum, midbrain, hypothalamus, thalamus, and brainstem are recommended. A comprehensive schematic diagram (see **Fig. 2** in Ref.[23]) is available for planning such sampling.[23] Obtaining these samples and starting the fixation process in the field or at the clinic before shipping can speed up diagnostic results (and minimize autolysis) as the laboratory will not have to wait for tissues to fix that were submitted fresh. However, in cases where rabies is a concern, sending the entire brain and brainstem fresh may be preferred by some laboratories. Multiple samples from different locations within the cerebral cortex should be collected as many diseases can be multifocal or "patchy," especially PEM, TME, and protozoal encephalitis. Necropsy and histopathology are critical to confirm the suspicion of PEM, for which the visible and microscopic lesions are localized in the gray matter of the cerebral cortex. For PEM, it is advantageous to specifically target the dorsal surfaces of the hemispheres, gather a sample in the caudal aspects of the hemispheres where PEM lesions tend to be more extensive, and adequately capture the junction between the white and gray matter.[24] The lesion of PEM is not etiologically specific, so unless there are lesions in other organ suggestive of cause (as might happen with lead intoxication), histopathology is not helpful in establishing a definitive etiology. The brain lesions of *H somni* are also often in the cerebral cortex, multifocal, and may be macroscopically localized. In the right clinical context, histopathology provides support for *H somni* diagnosis in the face of negative bacterial culture results (either from antimicrobial treatment or due to the multifocal distribution of lesions) as the vasculitis with thrombosis, inflammation, and hemorrhage are rather distinctive. This is also true for listeriosis (*Listeria monocytogenes*), which localizes to the brainstem, especially the pons and medulla, producing characteristic microabscesses.[24] An example of this characteristic histologic lesion is shown in **Fig. 9**. Failing to include the affected brainstem area in diagnostic samples can lead to a missed diagnosis. Listeriosis is traditionally associated

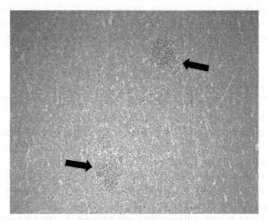

Fig. 9. H&E, 100X. Rhombencephalitis in a 5-year-old cow due to *L monocytogenes*. There are two small foci of inflammation (*arrows*) characterized by mostly neutrophils with fewer lymphocytes and glial cells mixed with karyorrhectic debris. The so-called "microabscesses" present within the bovine brainstem are virtually pathognomonic for listeriosis. (Photomicrograph courtesy of Matthew M. Hille.)

with animals being fed silage, but a recent report of rhombencephalitis caused by *L monocytogenes* in a bull on pasture suggests it should be included as a differential diagnosis in cases of neurologic disease even in the absence of silage feeding.[25]

Lesion patterns

As with other tissues, histopathology of the brain is important to establish the lesion reaction pattern (predominant cell type and microscopic location of the lesion such as perivascular vs meningeal, and so forth) to guide further testing. A few diseases with distinctive lesions have been mentioned, but it is important to understand the value and limitations to a pathologist identifying a reaction pattern with potentially several etiologies, especially nonsuppurative encephalitis. Purulent or fibrinous inflammation of the nervous system implies bacterial infection, and fungal lesions are often conspicuous with granulomatous inflammation and fungal elements visualized in the tissue. Nonsuppurative inflammation of the central nervous system is typically identified with a distinctive set of lesions: degeneration of neurons, perivascular cuffing by mononuclear cells (usually lymphocytes and plasma cells), and areas of glial proliferation (gliosis).[24] A diagnosis of nonsuppurative encephalitis will typically initiate a differential etiology list topped with viral causes, but certainly protozoa (*Neospora*), some bacterial infections, and neurodegeneration can elicit similar tissue changes. The diagnostician will attempt to identify anything distinctive about the lesion distribution and composition, particularly looking for the presence of features like viral inclusion bodies or necrotic foci with protozoal tachyzoites. Ancillary diagnostic tests may include specific tests for etiologies suited to the clinical history and any disease of high consequence, such as rabies. In the event that histopathology is poorly specific and advanced diagnostic testing detects no agent, there is little recourse other than to deem the case idiopathic or cause unknown.

Autolysis and decomposition pose a specific problem in the central nervous system in that it can obscure or mimic subtle degenerative change to the neuronal parenchyma. Even with substantial decomposition, it is possible to identify inflammatory diseases, like widespread meningoencephalitis. Autolysis and rough tissue handling can precipitate vacuolation which must be distinguished from spongy state.[26] The cellular constituents of the brain will begin to break down, and their cytological features and staining quality may change. Inadequate fixation may lead to a blurring of structural detail in histological sections.[26] Even if autolysis is unavoidable, it is helpful to follow standard principles of fixation to best preserve the tissue.

Hepatic Disease

The liver has a central role in the biological functions and systems-wide health of the animal. The pattern of cell death, inflammation, cellular adaptation, and/or tissue proliferation are important parameters used to formulate differential etiologies for liver injury and provide context for animals with a variety of clinical signs and complementary disease processes. For example, the brain lesions of hepatic encephalopathy could be overlooked but examination of a liver section could make the diagnosis more certain. The list of differential etiologies for liver disease can be extensive if the lesion is long-standing and without specific histologic changes and/or a detailed clinical history (as with chronic hepatitis terminating in cirrhosis). Other times, the diagnosis is more apparent, such as with multifocal hepatic necrosis and viral inclusions of bovine herpesvirus 1 abortion cases. The identification of lesions can depend on how diffuse and/or severe the changes are, that is, random liver biopsy is most useful for diffuse hepatopathies. The thorough postmortem examination would include "bread loafing," or serially sectioning, the entire liver parenchyma to evaluate for multifocal lesions to target in sample collection (a common example is liver abscesses). In some diseases (*Fascioloides magna, Clostridium novyi, Clostridium haemolyticum*), gross liver lesions are often unique and provide strong clinical etiologic evidence that can be confirmed in the laboratory using the sample collection guidelines described above.

Diffuse hepatopathies

A fine reticular pattern or random pale foci through the liver parenchyma at necropsy can often be seen, but histologic evaluation is necessary to differentiate common terminal vascular congestion from zonal necrosis and decomposition from random necrosis, respectively. Centrilobular necrosis is a common zonal pattern of hepatic necrosis and can be induced by intoxication or hypoxia. It may be unimportant to the primary cause of death in animals that have had a relatively chronic disease process before death with slowly failing circulation resulting in organ hypoxia. This may be supported by lesions in other organs such as kidney. Centrilobular necrosis may indicate cardiovascular failure, anemia (common with acute anaplasmosis), severe respiratory compromise, or hepatotoxins, but confirmation usually requires additional clinical or pathological information. Those cases with zonal necrosis suspected the result of a toxin often require additional clinical input and diagnostic investigation. Macroscopically, nonspecific centrilobular congestion may appear similar to necrotic change and histopathology can differentiate them. Random multifocal necrotizing hepatitis in the liver is a frequent pattern of injury which most commonly would have a bacterial or viral cause, often bacterial septicemia. It is also frequently seen in animals dying from various primary causes and not associated with a single agent bacterial septicemia, but rather is thought to be caused by bacteria breaching the gut mucosa barrier and reaching the liver through the splanchnic circulation. Frequently at necropsy, random pale areas in the liver are also created by localized colonies of saprophytic bacteria with accelerated tissue decomposition compared with the surrounding parenchyma. These examples show that changes in the liver are best evaluated with clear clinical context and histopathology of other organ systems and that common perimortem changes and decomposition can create the illusion of lesions which require histopathological confirmation.

Enteric Disease

Disease of the gastrointestinal can be associated with typical clinical observations such as diarrhea, dehydration, and/or abdominal bloating, or manifests as unexpected death without record of clinical signs. Outbreaks of enteric disease often have a complex multifactorial clinical picture (ie, failure of passive transfer and rapid dietary changes) to consider and incorporate with planning diagnostic evaluation. Histopathology is critical to demonstrating the disease agent associated with clinically relevant lesions, establishing the pattern of enteric injury, and sorting out the importance of ancillary diagnostic test results. This is especially true with the application of molecular panel testing, where samples are screened with high sensitivity for several disease agents at a time, many of which can be found at low levels even in healthy tissues.

Common problems that limit the value of histopathology in the gastrointestinal tract are poorly representative samples and postmortem changes. For the intestine, it is ideal to take several samples for fixation, representing the anatomical areas of duodenum, jejunum, ileum, colon, and cecum. Multiple samples of forestomach and abomasum may be required if this is of high clinical concern in the disease syndrome observed. It can be challenging to locate lesions during postmortem examination in adult cattle, as the intestine is roughly 33 to 63 m in length and can be challenging to manipulate.[27] Therefore, sampling is focused on the distal small intestine and colon, where lesions are most often observed. The diagnostic value of the large intestine is often overlooked, but coccidiosis and enteric coronavirus may manifest in their full impact on the colonic mucosa and the lesions can missed if only small intestine is viewed.[28,29] Another frequent occurrence is mistaking severely congested segments of the small intestine containing bloody, autolytic fluid for a lesion (hemorrhagic enteritis), and focusing sampling on this feature. Vascular congestion can occur around the time of death and, as autolysis proceeds, blood begins to leak from the deteriorating vessels. The evaluator should look for fibrin in the bloody intestinal content, mucosal ulcers, diphtheritic membranes, and/or edema to verify there is an inflammatory process present, and sample other tissues and areas of the intestine for thoroughness. Autolysis and decomposition introduce tissue artifacts that begin to develop in the mucosa of the gastrointestinal tract within minutes after death, first by exfoliation of the epithelial cells from the mucosal surface, which can also be an abnormal finding in the absence of autolysis.[30] Given that the rate artifacts form depends on many factors, it is difficult to estimate how long after death histopathology of the intestine loses its value, which would also likely vary depending on the disease and lesion severity. Although the experienced pathologist can "read through" autolytic change, it should be kept in mind that loss of the epithelium and distortion of the mucosa can mimic or mask important lesions.

Frequently, normal or incidental flora must be distinguished from a pathogen in enteric cases. This is particularly true with bacteria like *Escherichia coli* (*E coli*) and *Clostridium perfringens* (*Cl perfringens*). Histopathology is important to demonstrate the *E coli* virulence trait of bacterial colonization or adhesion to the mucosal surface of the intestine, particularly for the enterotoxigenic and enteropathogenic disease forms. *E coli* attachment to the apical surface of enterocytes may still be visible even with autolytic change where the enterocytes have exfoliated into the intestinal lumen, although tissue distortion and postmortem bacterial overgrowth in the intestinal lumen can obscure it over time. Finding this lesion may prompt scrutiny of bacterial culture isolates or give enough presumptive information on its own for clinical decisions. Histopathology is an important tool to discern the importance of *Cl perfringens* isolated from the gastrointestinal tract and guide further testing, particularly with the isolation of *Cl perfringens* type A, which can be found in the intestine of clinically normal cattle or those with intestinal disease and can overgrow in the intestinal lumen postmortem. Microscopic changes of mucosal hemorrhage, edema, inflammation, and evidence of mucosal injury like epithelial cell necrosis give support to the suspicion that the isolate is disease-causing.[31] In animals dying very quickly, and with early-stage lesions, postmortem autolysis and decomposition can easily obscure mucosal lesions and leave the isolation of *Cl perfringens* type A from the tissue difficult to interpret. A recent article provides excellent information on the clinical management of *Clostridial* abomasitis and enteritis.[32]

Abortions

Ruminant abortion investigations can be challenging as the likelihood of obtaining an etiologic diagnosis in an abortion outbreak is usually lower than other ruminant disease processes. Two retrospective studies from diagnostic laboratories in California and South Dakota showed an infectious etiologic diagnosis was confirmed in only 46.9% and 30.4% of cases respectively.[33,34] In the California study, bacterial culture of abomasal samples proved more sensitive than lung or liver. Cases that had lesions consistent with an infectious process, yet were negative using ancillary tests such as culture or molecular methods of pathogen detection, represented 11.7% and 17.34%

of diagnostic cases in California and South Dakota, respectively. The fact that histo-pathology was able to detect lesions suggestive of an infectious process when other methods failed, indicates the important role of the technique in abortion investigations. A histological examination is important to determine if there is evidence of infection in the absence of a confirmatory ancillary test. In addition, a lack of microscopic lesions suggestive of an infectious process can be valuable information clinically. In some cases, however, histopathology alone is able to confirm an etiologic diagnosis (**Fig. 10**).

The low diagnostic success rate in ruminant abortion cases is due to a number of causes. Fetuses can be retained by the dam for an extended period of time, resulting in severe postmortem autolysis of the fetal tissues. Although, even severely autolyzed fetal tissues can display characteristic histologic lesions to help guide or confirm a diagnosis in some circumstances (**Fig. 11**). Secondly, the placenta is a tissue that is important in ruling in or out the likelihood of an infectious process histologically yet is often not available for submission for a number of reasons.

A recent study that used both histopathology and molecular techniques to study normal bovine placentas had several interesting findings that highlight the need for diagnostic disease investigations to use all methods available, and interpret the results in total, and in clinical context. In that study, 20% of cotyledons were positive for *Coxiella burnetii* via PCR without microscopic evidence of an infectious process suggesting they were subclinical infections.[35] In addition, 20% of the clinically normal cotyledons examined exhibited inflammation and vasculitis. Therefore, the difficulty in determining the significance of one or two individual lesions can be problematic. Submitting more than one cotyledon for examination can help confirm a pattern.

Beyond just confirming the presence or absence of lesions associated with infectious processes, histopathology can help determine in full or near-full-term fetuses whether or not the case represents a true abortion (an expelled fetus before full term), a stillbirth (an expelled fetus at or very near term), or a perinatal death that was incorrectly assumed to be an abortion by the producer. A histologic examination can determine whether alveoli have previously expanded and identify excessive meconium in the lungs. A large amount of meconium within the lungs can indicate fetal

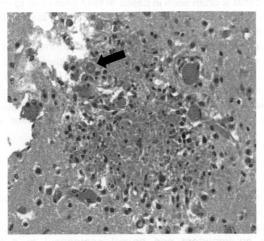

Fig. 10. H&E, 400X. Ovine protozoal abortion. Within the brain, there are multiple foci of necrosis surrounded by inflammatory cells. At the periphery of this necrotic focus, there is a protozoal cyst approximately 20 μm in diameter (*arrow*) consistent with ovine abortion due to *Toxoplasma* species of protozoa. (Photomicrograph courtesy of Matthew M. Hille.)

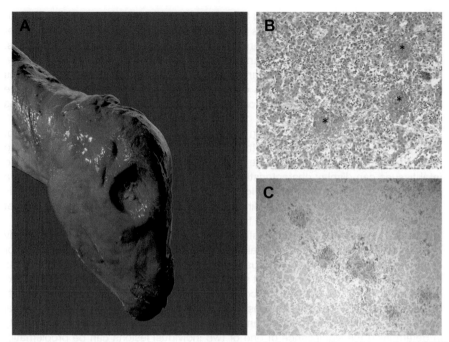

Fig. 11. Bovine abortion due to bovine herpesvirus-1 (infectious bovine rhinotracheitis [IBR] virus). (*A*) The aborted fetus was partially mummified with sunken eyes and marked autolysis of all tissues examined. (*B*) H&E, 100X. Despite the advanced autolytic changes in the liver, multiple foci of necrosis are still easily observed throughout the section (*asterisks*). (*C*) IBR immunohistochemistry (IHC), 100X. Abundant IBR antigen (*red* chromogen stain) is present within the necrotic foci. (Photograph and photomicrographs courtesy of Matthew M. Hille.)

stress, something that is often seen in cases of fetal death due to prolonged dystocia. Such information is important clinically to determine herd-level risk. It is important to note that due to the difficulties discussed above in investigation ruminant abortions, if a diagnosis is the goal, it requires a concerted effort on the part of the producer, the referring veterinarian, and the diagnostician, and a detailed clinical history.

A detailed discussion of individual causes of abortion in ruminants can be found in a previous veterinary clinics north america (VCNA) article which provides a good summary of the different causes of bovine abortion, specimens to submit, and how the different testing modalities can be leveraged to promote efficient abortion investigations.[36]

SUMMARY

The increasingly rapid technological advancements in diagnostic veterinary medicine make it an exciting time to investigate ruminant diseases. Newer techniques have undoubtedly increased the sensitivity and efficiency of diagnostic medicine, but histopathology remains an important and crucial component to a thorough disease investigation. Isolation of an agent in the context of a lesion remains the gold standard for assigning an etiologic diagnosis. The goal of this article was to briefly discuss some of the more common ruminant diseases that the authors' rely heavily on histopathology for a diagnosis and to discuss clinical techniques that can increase the likelihood of a successful diagnosis. The most common problem the authors' see in ruminant case submissions pertaining to histopathology is a lack of fixed tissue samples to examine. It is good practice to at least obtain fixed samples during routine necropsies. If the extra cost of histopathology beyond culture and/or PCR testing is a concern, the fixed tissues can be held by the diagnostic laboratory and only processed if deemed clinically indicated if ancillary testing is inconclusive.

CLINICS CARE POINTS

- Proper fixation and appropriate tissue handling preserves microscopic morphology leading to a more efficient histopathologic examination.

- A routine set of tissues should be obtained from all necropsies. Tissues can be examined on an "as needed" basis to minimize cost if that is a concern. Some laboratories charge a fee per specimen, whereas others do so only after a certain number of specimens has been reached. Become familiar with your laboratory's fee structure to maximize sample submission and diagnoses.

- If turnaround time is not particularly important for a given case, specimens can be fixed in the clinic for 24 to 36 hours and then shipped with just enough formalin to keep the tissues wet. Doing so provides adequate tissue fixation while minimizing the costs associated with shipping large jars of formalin.

- In cases of respiratory disease, sampling obvious gross lesions as well as adjacent, normal appearing tissue can help determine the disease process.

- The papillary muscle is the tissue of choice for suspected cases of histophilosis and ionophore toxicosis.

- Including placenta in an abortion investigation increases the likelihood of a definitive diagnosis.

ACKNOWLEDGMENTS

The authors would like to thank Scott Fritz for sharing images of gross lesions and Marcia Oetjen for her assistance with preparing gross images for publication.

DISCLOSURE

The authors have nothing to disclose.

REFERENCES

1. Steicke M, Yang G, Dinh TN, et al. The penetration of methanol into bovine cardiac and hepatic tissues is faster than ethanol and formalin. Eur J Histochem 2018;62(1):2880.
2. Robbins and cotran pathologic basis of disease. Tenth ed. Philadelphia: Elsevier Saunders; 2021.
3. Pathologic basis of veterinary disease. 6th ed. St. louis, MO: Elsevier; 2017.
4. Ensley S. Ionophore use and toxicosis in cattle. Vet Clin North Am Food Anim Pract 2020;36(3):641–52.
5. Booker CW, Abutarbush SM, Morley PS, et al. Microbiological and histopathological findings in cases of fatal bovine respiratory disease of feedlot cattle in Western Canada. Can Vet J 2008;49(5):473–81.

6. Uribe JA, Coura F, Nunes P, et al. Septicemic salmonellosis in pre weaned calves caused by Salmonella dublin. Res J Vet Pract 2015;3:69–75.

7. Loy JD, Leger L, Workman AM, et al. Development of a multiplex real-time PCR assay using two thermocycling platforms for detection of major bacterial pathogens associated with bovine respiratory disease complex from clinical samples. J Vet Diagn Invest 2018;30(6):837–47.

8. Thonur L, Maley M, Gilray J, et al. One-step multiplex real time RT-PCR for the detection of bovine respiratory syncytial virus, bovine herpesvirus 1 and bovine parainfluenza virus 3. BMC Vet Res 2012;8(1):37.

9. Woolums AR. Feedlot acute interstitial pneumonia. Vet Clin North Am Food Anim Pract 2015;31(3):381–9.

10. Blood D. Atypical interstitial pneumonia of cattle. Can Vet J 1962;2:40–7.

11. Doster AR. Bovine atypical interstitial pneumonia. Vet Clin North Am Food Anim Pract 2010;26(2):395–407.

12. Galitzer SJ, Kruckenberg SM, Kidd JR. Pathologic changes associated with experimental lasalocid and monensin toxicosis in cattle. Am J Vet Res 1986; 47(12):2624–6.

13. Hudson LM, Kerr LA, Maslin WR. Gossypol toxicosis in a herd of beef calves. J Am Vet Med Assoc 1988;192(9):1303–5.

14. Barth AT, Kommers GD, Salles MS, et al. Coffee senna (senna occidentalis) poisoning in cattle in Brazil. Vet Hum Toxicol 1994;36(6):541–5.

15. Calò M, Lo Cascio P, Licata P, et al. Effects of monensin on Na+/K(+)-ATPase and Ca(++)-AtPase activities in chick skeletal muscle and myocardium after subacute treatment. Eur J Histochem 2002;46(4):309–15.

16. O'Toole D, Sondgeroth KS. Histophilosis as a natural disease. Curr Top Microbiol Immunol 2016;396:15–48.

17. Welsh RD, Dye LB, Payton ME, et al. Isolation and antimicrobial susceptibilities of bacterial pathogens from bovine pneumonia: 1994–2002. J Vet Diagn Invest 2004;16(5):426–31.

18. Margineda CA, O'Toole D, Prieto M, et al. Histophilus somni myocarditis and leptomeningitis in feedlot cattle: case report and occurrence in South America. J Vet Diagn Invest 2019;31(6):893–8.

19. Headley SA, Voltarelli D, de Oliveira VH, et al. Association of Histophilus somni with spontaneous abortions in dairy cattle herds from Brazil. Trop Anim Health Prod 2015;47(2):403–13.

20. Madampage CA, Rawlyk N, Crockford G, et al. Single nucleotide polymorphisms in the bovine Histophilus somni genome; a comparison of new and old isolates. Can J Vet Res 2015;79(3):190–200.

21. Capik SF, Moberly HK, Larson RL. Systematic review of vaccine efficacy against Mannheimia haemolytica, Pasteurella multocida, and Histophilus somni in North American cattle. Bovine Pract 2021;55(2):125–33.

22. Griffin D. Field necropsy of cattle and diagnostic sample submission. Vet Clin North Am Food Anim Pract 2012;28(3):391–405.

23. Rech R, Giaretta PR, Brown C, et al. Gross and histopathological pitfalls found in the examination of 3,338 cattle brains submitted to the BSE surveillance program in Brazil. Pesquisa Veterinaria Brasileira 2018;38(11):2099–108.

24. Maxie MG. Jubb, Kennedy, and Palmer's pathology of domestic animals. 6th. edition. Amsterdam, Netherlands: Elsevier; 2016.

25. Matto C, Varela G, Mota M, et al. Rhombencephalitis caused by Listeria monocytogenes in a pastured bull. J Vet Diagn Invest 2017;29. 104063871668911.

26. Vandevelde M, Higgins RJ, Overmann A. Veterinary neuropathology : essentials of theory and practice. Oxford: Wiley-Blackwell; 2012.
27. Sreekanth C, Shakuntala Rao N, Manivannan K, et al. Caecum and appendix in ruminants and man: a comparative study. J Evol Med Dental Sci 2014;3:8033–9.
28. Stockdale PH. The pathogenesis of the lesions produced by Eimeria zuernii in calves. Can J Comp Med 1977;41(3):338–44.
29. Boileau MJ, Kapil S. Bovine coronavirus associated syndromes. Vet Clin North Am Food Anim Pract 2010;26(1):123–46.
30. Pearson GR, Logan EF. The rate of development of postmortem artefact in the small intestine of neonatal calves. Br J Exp Pathol 1978;59(2):178–82.
31. Goossens E, Valgaeren BR, Pardon B, et al. Rethinking the role of alpha toxin in Clostridium perfringens-associated enteric diseases: a review on bovine necro-haemorrhagic enteritis. Vet Res 2017;48(1):9.
32. Simpson KM, Callan RJ, Van Metre DC. Clostridial abomasitis and enteritis in ruminants. Vet Clin North Am Food Anim Pract 2018;34(1):155–84.
33. Clothier K, Anderson M. Evaluation of bovine abortion cases and tissue suitability for identification of infectious agents in California diagnostic laboratory cases from 2007 to 2012. Theriogenology 2016;85(5):933–8.
34. Kirkbride CA. Etiologic agents detected in a 10-year study of bovine abortions and stillbirths. J Vet Diagn Invest 1992;4(2):175–80.
35. Botta C, Pellegrini G, Hässig M, et al. Bovine fetal placenta during pregnancy and the postpartum period. Vet Pathol 2019;56(2):248–58.
36. Holler LD. Ruminant abortion diagnostics. Vet Clin North Am Food Anim Pract 2012;28(3):407–18.

Current and Emerging Diagnostic Approaches to Bacterial Diseases of Ruminants

John Dustin Loy, DVM, PhD, DACVM[a],*, Michael L. Clawson, PhD[b],
Pamela R.F. Adkins, DVM, PhD, DACVIM (LAIM)[c],
John R. Middleton, DVM, PhD, DACVIM (LAIM)[c]

KEYWORDS

- Bovine • Diagnostics • Bacterial pathogens • MALDI-TOF • Real-time PCR
- Bovine respiratory disease • Mastitis • Abortion • Bovine keratoconjunctivitis

KEY POINTS

- Real-time polymerase chain reaction (PCR) methods have enabled highly sensitive diagnostic tests for numerous bacterial pathogens of ruminants.
- Multiplexing of real-time PCR tests has enabled development of syndromic PCR panels that can screen for several pathogens in one test.
- Real-time PCR cycle threshold values can be used to estimate relative abundance of pathogens in clinical samples.
- Comparison of molecular diagnostics with culture-based approaches is disease- and sample-dependent.
- Matrix-assisted laser desorption ionization–time-of-flight mass spectrometry has allowed for highly efficient identification and typing of bacterial pathogens associated with ruminant diseases.

INTRODUCTION
Basics of Polymerase Chain Reaction

The polymerase chain reaction (PCR) was discovered in the mid-1980s and remains one of the most important developments to molecular biology.[1] Specifically, the adaptation of this technique to use with fluorescent dyes and labeled probes, allowing measurement of nucleic acid amplification in real time, the real-time PCR (rtPCR) assay

[a] Nebraska Veterinary Diagnostic Center, School of Veterinary Medicine and Biomedical Sciences, University of Nebraska-Lincoln, Lincoln, NE, USA; [b] USDA, Agriculture Research Service US Meat Animal Research Center, Clay Center, NE, USA; [c] Department of Veterinary Medicine and Surgery, College of Veterinary Medicine, University of Missouri, Columbia, MO, USA
* Corresponding author. Nebraska Veterinary Diagnostic Center, University of Nebraska-Lincoln, Lincoln, 4040 East Campus Loop N., Lincoln, NE 68583-0907.
E-mail address: jdloy@unl.edu

Vet Clin Food Anim 39 (2023) 93–114
https://doi.org/10.1016/j.cvfa.2022.10.006
0749-0720/23/© 2022 Elsevier Inc. All rights reserved.

has had the greatest impact in veterinary diagnostic laboratories (VDLs).[2] The acronym rtPCR will be used throughout this article to describe this approach as has been used in a recent review on this method specific to VDLs.[2] Other nomenclature or acronyms to describe similar methods for RNA detection include reverse transcription rtPCR (RT-rtPCR). The acronyms qPCR and RT-qPCR are recommended for use by the *Minimum Information for Publication of Quantitative Real-Time PCR Experiments* guidelines, so these are frequently used to describe rtPCR and RT-rtPCR in the literature.[3] However, this convention is not applied in this review, as qPCR implies quantification of target, which does not routinely occur when used for diagnostic testing. rtPCR applied to diagnostic testing of veterinary samples is complex and includes collection and transport of samples, sample preparation, nucleic acid extraction, amplification, analysis, and reporting. One advantage of rtPCR is there is no additional step required to visualize amplification, which decreases analysis time and reduces risk for cross-contamination, as amplified targets do not need additional processing or handling. The extreme sensitivity of the method, which can detect a few nucleic acid copies, requires strict quality control to ensure accuracy.

The rtPCR methods have been developed for detection of numerous pathogens, many of which are multiplexed assays that allow for simultaneous testing for multiple targets in the same sample.[4] Multiplexing typically relies on the use of sequence specific oligonucleotides, called probes, that have a reporter dye and quencher dye attached to the 5′ and 3′ end, and are combined in an assay with flanking oligonucleotide primers. During nucleic acid amplification the reporter and quencher dyes are cleaved from the probe by the polymerase enzyme, resulting in fluorescence of the reporter dye when excited by the light source from the instrument. Numerous reporter dyes are available that can be multiplexed as they differ in their emission spectrum following excitation. This has allowed for the development of syndrome specific panels (syndromic PCR panels) that allow for rapid screening of numerous agents associated with a disease syndrome. The real-time nature of the assay allows for fluorescence to be measured following each amplification cycle (typically 40 total cycles; **Figs. 1** and **2**). The number of cycles required to generate sufficient signal over background levels is called a cycle threshold (Ct) value, which is inversely proportional to the amount of target in the sample. This relationship allows for quantification of target in the sample to be conducted by comparison with a standard curve of a known and quantified target, also called a cycle quantification (Cq) level (see **Fig. 1**). However, the use of a standard curve for quantification is cost and time prohibitive and typically not

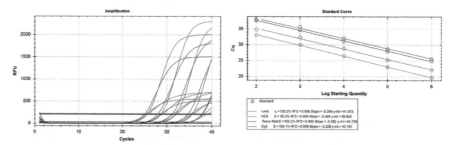

Fig. 1. Real-time PCR amplification plots demonstrating use of four targets in a serial dilution. X-axis is cycles and y-axis is relative fluorescence (*left panel*) and a generation of a standard curve from these data, x-axis is cycle threshold (Ct) value and y-axis is log-starting quantity of target (*right panel*). The increase in Ct value for each serial dilution can be observed, along with relative differences in values for each target.

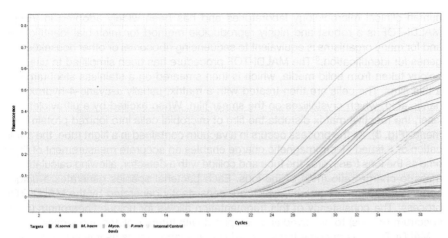

Fig. 2. Real-time PCR data output showing baseline corrected fluorescence in a multiplexed rtPCR panel for bovine respiratory disease run on clinical samples. Each colored line on the curve represents a single target (*H somni*, *M haemolytica*, *P multocida*, *M bovis*, and Internal Control) within the multiplexed reaction run on nucleic acid extracted from a sample.

performed for routine diagnostics (see note above about rtPCR and qPCR). Instead, the Ct value is used and reported based on the relative abundance of target in comparison to a well characterized positive control. VDLs typically report this on diagnostic reports as a Ct value and have established cutoffs to determine if a sample is considered detected (positive) for a target, or not detected (negative) based on their validation studies. These components are necessary for Ct values to be meaningful in the absence of a standard curve.[2] Therefore, in this article, Ct value will be used instead of Cq or other metrics, as this is the most commonly reported on diagnostic results.

Diagnostic applications of rtPCR using multiplexing have expanded the range of agents available for testing, simplified reporting, and reduced testing costs. There are some limitations, however, because robust optimization must be undertaken to ensure no preferential target amplification is occurring. This can cause false-negative results for some low-copy targets when amplified in the presence of a strong positive, a frequent occurrence for some disease syndromes such as bacteria associated with bovine respiratory disease (BRD).[4,5] To ensure consistent assay performance, VDLs will typically include a low-copy internal positive control (IPC) which is an exogenous source of nucleic acid that can be measured to ensure no inhibitors are present in the sample and that the nucleic acid extraction performed as expected.[6] IPCs are also useful to evaluate the presence of preferential amplification in multiplexed assays, as amplification of the low-copy control can be evaluated to ensure this is not occurring.

Expanded development, validation, and accessibility of rtPCR have made numerous tests for ruminant diagnostics available in VDLs. Research continues to provide meaningful data in associating these test results to both classical tests and field-level investigations. Specific discussion of these tests is provided later in this article using frequently encountered clinical disease syndromes of ruminants.

Matrix-Assisted Laser Desorption Ionization–Time of Flight and Diagnostics

Matrix-assisted laser desorption ionization–time-of-flight (MALDI-TOF) mass spectrometry is an emerging technology that has revolutionized bacterial identification in human clinical microbiology laboratories and has been widely adopted in VDLs.[7] MALDI-TOF is a robust and highly reproducible method for microbial identification and for many organisms is equivalent to sequencing ribosomal or other housekeeping genes for identification.[8] The MALDI-TOF procedure has been simplified to use on a colony taken from solid media, which is then smeared on a stainless steel target in a thin film.[9] The cells are then treated with a matrix, usually α-cyano-4-hydroxycinnamic acid, which crystallizes on the smear film. When excited by a ultraviolet (UV) laser, the reactive matrix disrupts the film of microbial cells into ionized protein fragments (**Fig. 3**). As the process occurs in a vacuum contained in a flight tube, the application of a timed electromagnetic charge enables an accurate measurement of flight time as the ions transverse the tube and collide with a detector, allowing calculation of mass-to-charge ratio (m/z) of the ions. Each bacterial species generates a unique composition of ion fragments, which are consistently generated by the MALDI-TOF process. The consistency of this fragmentation allows for unique fingerprints (mass spectrum profiles) to be saved and compared with future isolates and strains.

MALDI-TOF has become the standard in many laboratories as it is fast, reproducible, cost-efficient, accurate, and eliminates the need for specialized biochemical testing. Commercially available MALDI-TOF libraries have tens of thousands of database entries; some of which include yeasts and molds in addition to human, veterinary, plant, and environmental bacterial pathogens and organisms. Studies have been conducted examining this technology for many veterinary and bovine pathogens including those associated with mastitis, respiratory disease, and ocular disease.[10–13] Laboratories can also curate their own database of profiles for isolates or strains that may be more regional, disease, or host-specific.[11] In addition, methods have been developed that enable discrimination of specific peaks contained in the mass spectrum profile that can be used to characterize isolates to the subspecies level, which may be useful when culturing opportunistic pathogens from sites with normal flora.[14–16] Many instruments also possesses the ability for biotyping, or looking at relatedness dendrograms based on peak profiles, which may be useful for outbreak investigations or evaluating strain diversity in herds or regions for some pathogens.[17]

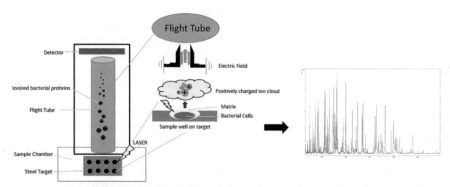

Fig. 3. Diagram of MALDI-TOF process for microbial identification. A thin film of microbial cells is prepared with a matrix solution on a steel target. The sample is vaporized into positively charged ions by a laser, which are propelled through a vacuum flight tube by an electrical field. Ions hitting the detector are measured and mass to charge ratio (m/z) is calculated. Mass spectrum output is shown next to the black arrow. Blue is *M bovis* and red is *M bovoculi*. The x-axis is m/z in Daltons. The y-axis is peak intensity in arbitrary units (arbitrary units). The mass spectrum profiles generated can then be used for downstream identification or strain typing.

Basics of Sequencing for Identification

Identification of bacterial pathogens can be challenging, even with robust tools such as MALDI-TOF, PCR, and gene sequencing. Bacterial genomes typically consist of a circular chromosome, and in some cases, plasmids or phages can be fluid.[18–20] Bacteria can acquire exogenous deoxyribonucleic acid (DNA) through plasmid- or integrative conjugative element (ICE)- induced conjugation, viral-induced transduction, and transformation processes, which collectively result in plasmid acquisitions, and the assimilation of ICEs and other newly acquired DNA segments on to their chromosomes.[21] In addition, insertion sequences and larger transposons can move about bacterial DNA,[21,22] so too can integrons, which are assembly and expression platforms of exogenous gene cassettes that can reside on plasmids and transposons where they have mobility.[23] Bacterial chromosomes and plasmids can also change their tandem repeat numbers due to strand slippage and recombination, and they can undergo inversions.[24–26] Bacteria also have mutation rates with their reproduction that can vary within a community and result in the spontaneous generation of single nucleotide polymorphisms and/or insertion deletion alleles.[27,28] All of these mechanisms can introduce or modulate gene function in bacteria, and thus are essential to their evolution and adaptability to new niches, including ones involving pathogenesis.[21,22,29] Consequently, decoding their genomic playbooks through sequencing provides a means for their identification and a foundation for understanding their biological functions and pathogenic potential.

DNA sequencing technology has advanced tremendously through the years and is categorized into three generations. The first is represented by Maxam–Gilbert and Sanger techniques that provide relatively small-scale sample and targeted region coverage.[30,31] The second consists of massive, short-length sequence production from clonally amplified DNA molecules on platforms such as Ion Torrent and Illumina.[30] The short-length sequences produced with second-generation technologies translate to challenges in generating compete, closed whole-genome assemblies, primarily because of repetitive sequence as well as genomic rearrangements and inversions.[30,32,33] Third-generation sequencing technologies involve moving a strand of DNA along a stationary read out system, such as an immobilized DNA polymerase complex (PacBio platform), or through a pore on a membrane, where ion flow changes through the membrane coincide with the nucleotides passing through it (Oxford Nanopore platform).[30] DNA sequence reads generated from third-generation technologies tend to be much longer than those from the second generation, which means that they assemble better; however, the sequence reads can have higher error rates.[30] Consequently, hybrid assemblies using combinations of second- and third-generation sequences have been used to generate highly accurate, closed bacterial chromosome sequences.[34] Third-generation sequencing continues to improve, and combined with enhanced assembly techniques, shows promise in constructing closed, circular genomes from mixed samples containing DNA of multiple microbes, such as microbiome samples.[35] Thus, the ability to sequence and assemble full bacterial chromosomes, even from preparations of mixed DNA, should only continue to increase in the future.

Nucleic acid sequence is a powerful identifier of bacteria. Historically, 16S ribosomal gene sequence has been used for bacterial identification to the species level.[36] More recently, its taxonomic utility has been recognized more at the level of genus or higher with only segments of the gene used for identification.[37,38] Multilocus sequence analysis, which involves analysis of multiple (4 or more) housekeeping genes, is commonly used for species and subspecies identification.[39] However, with whole-genome sequencing (WGS) of bacteria becoming cheaper, faster, and easier to do, average nucleotide identity (ANI) has become a preferred metric of choice for species identification.[40] The ANI method was developed in 2005 and is an alignment-based pairwise similarity between two genomes.[40–42] Bacterial genomes do not have to be completely assembled into single chromosomes for ANI comparisons, and simple cut-offs are used to determine if bacteria are members of the same species.[43,44] Thus, it has become somewhat straightforward to identify bacterial species. Whole genomic sequences can also be used to identify bacterial subspecies, usually by phylogenetic or cladistic analyses that show genetic substructure at that level.[34,45,46] As sequencing technologies continue to improve and become cheaper and more acces-sible, we anticipate that WGS will become increasingly used by VDLs for a variety of applications.

APPLICATION IN DIAGNOSING SPECIFIC CLINICAL SYNDROMES
Bovine Respiratory Disease

BRD is a multifactorial disease complex associated with both viruses and bacteria and is one of the most frequently diagnosed and economically costly diseases of cattle.[47] Bacterial pathogens associated with BRD include *Mannheimia haemolytica*, *Pasteur-ella multocida*, *Histophilus somni*, *Mycoplasma bovis*, and organisms such as *Trueper-ella pyogenes*.[47] Culture and downstream identification methods, such as biochemical testing, are the gold standard for diagnosis of bacterial pathogens associated with BRD. However, numerous molecular-based PCR assays are available for detection and identification of bacterial pathogens associated with BRD. The most efficient use highly multiplexed assays that can detect several pathogens in a single test and can be used on nasal swabs, bronchoalveolar lavage fluid, and lung tissues.[5,48–51] Similar approaches have been developed and implemented for viral BRD pathogens for more than a decade.[52] rtPCR for BRD pathogens has significant advantages in testing time and sensitivity; however, interpretation varies depending on the sample type and amount of potential contaminating flora, even in robustly validated assays as many of these pathogens are opportunists that can reside in the nasopharynx of normal animals (see a previous edition for a recent review of BRD clinical diagnostics and sampling).[53] Generally, PCR has been established as more sensitive at BRD path-ogen detection than culture, by as much as 20% in one study.[54] Another advantage to syndromic rtPCR panel-based approaches over conventional methods is the enhanced ability to identify co-detections. In one study, co-detection of BRD patho-gens were not observed when relying on culture alone but a five-fold increase in co-detections was observed using rtPCR.[5] The rtPCR also has advantages for detecting fastidious and slow growing agents like *Mycoplasma bovis*, where culture can take weeks and rtPCR is rapid and sensitive.[55] Many laboratories also include a culture-based diagnostic as part of the PCR panel to supplement recovery of isolates for downstream testing like antimicrobial susceptibility. Relating PCR results to culture and other traditional diagnostics is complex as the detection of target pathogen nucleic acid is not the same as isolation of a viable pathogen. The limitations for rtPCR-based diagnostics for BRD have been well discussed previously.[56] However, the use of Ct which is associated with relative pathogen abundance can be useful to estimate pathogen burden. For example, in BRD assays that were compared with culture, limits of detection for PCR were quite low (1.2–12 colony forming units [CFU]/mL), with Ct values ranging from ~36 to 37 for this level. Each subsequent decrease of 2 to 3 Ct corresponded to a 10-fold increase in copy number, thus providing some data for clinicians to use to support association of the relative amount of pathogen with the observed disease.[5]

Gaps still exist in objectively relating Ct values to clinical disease, especially with antemortem samples like nasal swabs. However, a recent study looked at pathogen Ct values detected in nasal swabs in relationship to BRD clinical scores to estimate clinically relevant Ct cutoffs. Although the cutoffs calculated are not directly comparable with other assays, because the method uses a pre-amplification step, it means that there are potentially clinically useful relationships between nasal swab pathogen shedding as detected by PCR and clinical BRD for some pathogens.[57]

Other applications for these tools are also being realized, such as examining the relationships between pathogen circulation and BRD outbreaks.[58,59] The rtPCR technology is also being applied to rapidly determine the presence of antimicrobial resistance genes and thus be able to assist therapy selection in near real time. One study showed high to moderate levels of agreement between isolation of resistant bacterial BRD pathogens and detection of macrolide or tetracycline resistance genes in clinical samples.[60] Third-generation sequencing tools are also being applied to look at both antimicrobial resistance and pathogen detection.[61]

Other emerging tools to rapidly identify and characterize pathogens from samples include the use of MALDI-TOF. Recent advantages allow for rapid genotyping of *M haemolytica* isolates to discern those types more likely to be associated with BRD, which is especially helpful when culturing samples like nasal swabs that may have mixed populations.[14,62] Other new methods include the use of MALDI-TOF to characterize tetracycline resistance and directly detect BRD pathogens from enriched clinical samples.[63,64]

Recent research highlights the advantages of multimodal BRD diagnostics, where PCR or molecular-based testing can be combined with classical culture-based approaches and even direct application of mass spectrometry to clinical samples to rapidly determine the presence or absence of agents associated with disease, estimate the relative pathogen burdens in complex samples, and provide some rudimentary assessment of the presence or absence of antimicrobial resistance before pathogen isolation. Given that pathogenicity within a bacterial species such as *M haemolytica* can vary at the strain level, isolates can be characterized by MALDI-TOF to determine if they are more or less likely to be a pathogen, before being subjected to MIC testing for antimicrobial resistance (AMR) phenotypes.

Infectious Bovine Keratoconjunctivitis

Like BRD, infectious bovine keratoconjunctivitis (IBK) is a disease complex, with numerous pathogens associated with the disease, each with varying degrees of support for causality. The IBK complex remains one of the most frequently reported diseases of cow–calf producers.[65] This subject was recently reviewed in a previous edition of Veterinary Clinics of North America (VCNA) dedicated to ruminant opthamology.[66,67] Typically, diagnostic testing includes detection and/or isolation of *Moraxella bovis, Moraxella bovoculi*, bovine herpesvirus-1 (Bo-HV1), and *Mycoplasma* spp. The use of flocked swabs in a liquid transport media is used to facilitate testing both by PCR panels and culture as many of these pathogens are intimately associated with epithelial cells.

Specific testing approaches for IBK are similar to BRD, where syndromic panels have been developed that can screen for relevant pathogens using rtPCR, and Ct values may be useful to estimate pathogen shedding.[68] Newer panels include repeats-in-toxin (RTX) gene targets for *M bovis* and *M bovoculi,* which may help support clinical relevance of detection. Culture is performed as a supplement to collect isolates for downstream testing such as autogenous vaccine manufacture and/or antimicrobial susceptibility testing.[69] However, in the authors' experience, the high rates of detection by rtPCR of some pathogens, especially *M bovis* and *Mycoplasma bovoculi*, do not associate with high rates of isolation by culture. This may be due to fastidiousness of the organisms, contaminating flora, or the rapid penetration of some strains into the cornea following infection.[70] Culture is also beneficial because *in vitro* multidrug resistance to the approved IBK therapies (tulathromycin and oxytetracycline) has been observed in some strains of *M bovoculi*, although not frequently in *M bovis*.[45,71]

MALDI-TOF has been used to develop rapid typing tools to discern genotypes of *M bovoculi* at the subspecies level. Thus, it can rapidly discriminate between one genotype associated with IBK and another more likely to be found in normal animals.[15] MALDI-TOF-based typing tools have also been developed to rapidly screen for isolates that carry hemolytic RTXs using supplemented agar media.[72]

Infectious Abortion

Infectious abortion in cattle can be caused by pathogenic bacteria, fungi, parasites, and viruses.[73] Although diagnosis of infectious abortion should rely heavily on histopathology (see Matthew M. Hille and colleagues' article, "The Role of Histopathology in Ruminant Diagnostics," in this issue), it can benefit from supplemental diagnostics such as culture, rtPCR, syndromic rtPCR panels, and even WGS of isolates. Infectious abortions in one study accounted for 58% of abortion cases submitted to one US diagnostic laboratory, so detection and/or identification of these agents is important.[74] It is also critical to determine if the cause of abortion may provide risk to other herdmates or is the result of an opportunistic infection. The most frequently encountered bacterial pathogens include *T pyogenes*, *Bacillus* spp, *Listeria* spp, *Leptospira* spp, and enterobacteria such as *Salmonella* and *Escherichia coli*.[73,75] Other US studies have also found *Campylobacter* spp in some cases.[74] Traditionally, classical diagnostics focused on culture-based approaches; however, PCR has advantages in speed and sensitivity. New technologies including fluorescent *in situ* hybridization and 16S ribosomal deoxyribonucleic acid (rDNA) sequencing have also shown improvement in detection of infectious agents, especially for fungi.[76] Tissues available and lesion types may guide testing. For example, placenta with histological evidence of placentitis benefits from PCR, because cultures are frequently contaminated and may have false-negative or false-positive culture results.[77] Placenta seems to be infrequently submitted, potentially due to placentophagia or scavenging (one study had inclusion in only 12.5% of submissions); however, it would be important for detection of *Chlamydia* and *Coxiella burnetii* if these agents are suspected.[74,78] Other tissues are generally less susceptible to contamination, so detections and/or recovery of infectious agents with consistent lesions may be more meaningful. One study showed fetal abomasum had the greatest likelihood of pathogen detection, so this would be useful to include in submissions for both culture and PCR testing.[74]

To supplement other diagnostics, multiplexed rtPCR assays have been developed that target a broad range of agents associated with bovine infectious abortion.[79] One challenge over other disease syndromes is the agents associated with bovine abortions vary greatly with management strategies and geographical and international boundaries and includes zoonotic pathogens. Many agents, such as *Brucella* spp are infrequent in the United States due to control programs, and therefore, the need for inclusion in routine diagnostic panels is limited. Another example is the foothill abortion agents, or epizootic bovine abortion, caused by *Pajaroellobacter abortibovis*, which is predominant in cases occurring where the agent is endemic.[74,80] Other laboratories in Europe report *Neospora* and *Bacillus licheniformis* as leading causes of infectious abortions, which may not be observed with the same frequency elsewhere.[77]

One study from Switzerland detected *C burnetii* in 20% of placentomes tested.[78] Currently, author Loy's laboratory uses a multiplex rtPCR panel that contains viral, bacterial, and parasitic causes of infectious abortion to supplement histopathology. These include bovine viral diarrhea virus, Bo-HV1, *Neospora caninum*, and *Leptospira* spp.[52,81–83] Even though it is not a bacterium, *Neospora* PCR is a helpful target to include in syndromic panels, as it remains a widespread issue in numerous herds and may not always induce lesions. A review of control and diagnosis of *Neospora* can be found in the earlier VCNA editions.[84]

WGS of isolates may also be a useful tool to investigate infectious abortion. A recent study examined a large abortion outbreak caused by *Listeria monocytogenes* using WGS to compare strains isolated from clinical cases and their environment, which identified two distinct strains isolated from the abortions, with one also found in water and silage sources. The origin of other strain was not idenitifed.[85] This highlights the potential impact of WGS to help identify and eliminate sources of pathogens associated with abortion in the environment.

Enteric Infections: Calf Diarrhea

Calf diarrhea is one of the most economically significant diseases in beef and dairy cattle and is estimated to cause more than half of calf mortality on dairy farms.[86] The most frequently identified pathogens associated with calf diarrhea (calves less than 30 days) include *Cryptosporidium*, rotavirus, bovine coronavirus, *Salmonella* spp, and pathogenic *E coli*.[87] Classically, these pathogens were diagnosed with a combination of methods including culture, histopathology (at postmortem), electron microscopy, and other methods such as an enzyme-linked immunosorbent assay (ELISA).[87] However, syndromic PCR panels have been developed which enable rapid screening for many of them using multiplexed rtPCR.[48,88] Other non-PCR-based rapid tests (antigen-capture ELISA dipsticks) are also available that screen for antigens of a similar array of pathogens; however, sensitivity, especially for viral agents may be decreased.[89] Additional information on detection and diagnosis of viral agents, including those associated with diarrhea is found in another article of this edition and in reviews including pathophysiology and treatments in earlier VCNA editions.[90]

For bacterial infections, such as *E coli*, the vast majority of organisms in the intestinal tract are commensals, and only a small percentage are pathogenic. Therefore, determining the causality of isolates recovered from clinical cases often requires the determination of the presence or absence of virulence factors. *E coli* is primarily associated with two enteric diseases in cattle, one being neonatal diarrhea primarily caused by enterotoxigenic *E coli* (ETEC) and another associated with Shiga toxin-producing *E coli*/attaching and effacing *E coli*.[91] For a comprehensive review of *E coli* associated with both attaching and effacing disease and calf diarrhea please see additional chapters in previous VCNA editions.[87,92] ETEC is the primary cause of neonatal diarrhea in the first 4 days of life.[86] However, determination of the presence of virulence factors is routinely conducted on isolates from clinical cases and can include PCR panels to determine the presence or absence of both toxins and adherence factors in bacterial isolates.[93] Direct detection of the *E coli* K99/F5 gene, which encodes a fimbrial antigen involved with adhesion, is usually included in syndromic panels run on fecal samples due to overlap in age and clinical presentation with other pathogens.[88] In some of the authors' experience, ETEC K99/F5 is readily detected by rtPCR when present, with a corresponding low Ct value and heavy growth of a mucoid isolate on selective agar when cultured.

Salmonellosis in calves 2 to 6 weeks of age can cause diarrhea and severe enteric disease with variable severity.[94] In adult cattle, acute forms of disease can be characterized by fever followed by diarrhea and abortions in pregnant animals.[94] Most clinical infections with *Salmonella* are caused by the host-adapted serotype Dublin in addition to Typhimurium.[94] However, a recent study reported more than 143 serotypes found in normal cattle, with the most frequent being Montevideo, Typhimurium, Kentucky, Meleagridis, Anatum, Cerro, Mbandaka, Muenster, Newport, and Senftenberg.[95] This indicates that multiple serotypes are circulating in cattle populations worldwide. *Salmonella* spp are routinely detectable by culture and samples from animals with fecal shedding levels of 100 CFU/gram or greater are readily detected, which is a level routinely found in clinical cases.[96] However, culture for *Salmonella* spp typically includes several enrichment and/or selection steps that take several days. Therefore, *Salmonella* is an ideal target for PCR panels and any detection should be considered significant. In the VDL of author Loy, laboratory culture testing is routinely performed on any nonnegative *Salmonella* PCR test from feces or tissues, and positive culture results are typically yielded in cases where Ct values are $\leq$ 35. Isolation of *Salmonella* following a culture-independent diagnostic test like PCR is an important reflex test to perform, as strains vary significantly in virulence depending on serotype and antimicrobial susceptibility testing may be requested. One diagnostic challenge is *Salmonella* Dublin, which can be shed at low levels and/or is intermittently shed and does not grow well on routine selective media. Thus, sensitivity in subclinical shedding animals is estimated to be 20%.[97] New methods of detection of very low levels of *Salmonella* are useful for environmental and testing of subclinical shedders that combine enrichment followed by PCR.[97] Serological tests using an indirect ELISA are available for *Salmonella* Dublin and may be helpful to determine previous or current infection or herd status.[98] Recent reviews of *Salmonella* in dairy cattle and calves can be found in previous VCNA editions.[99,100]

Enteric Infections: Johne's Disease

Johne's disease, caused by *Mycobacterium avium* ssp *paratuberculosis* (MAP), is an economically significant and widespread disease of ruminants worldwide. An excellent review of MAP diagnostics is provided in a previous VCNA edition, which states "There is a suitable diagnostic test for virtually every paratuberculosis need."[101] The gold standard diagnostic test is fecal culture; however, this is time-consuming, laborious, and very few VDLs currently offer it due to cost and time requirements. Most laboratories rely on rtPCR (typically insertion sequence 900) for MAP diagnostics in addition to serological testing for MAP antibodies. New testing methods using mycobacteriophage D29 have been developed that may enable enhanced diagnostic testing, as they only infect and lyse viable MAP cells; however, they need further validation to become commercially viable.[102] Consensus recommendations on MAP diagnostics have been developed by experts based on different animal production purposes, species, and systems.[103] Tests and test recommendations are frequently designed with control programs in mind and are extremely useful for determining herd-level status and risk. In addition to control programs, frequently diagnosticians and veterinarians are tasked with applying MAP diagnostics to individual valuable or seedstock animals, where the recommended test is typically fecal PCR. Interpretation of PCR results for MAP is usually straightforward, as the specificity of the test is greater than 95%, thus animals that are PCR positive are likely infected.[103,104] However, this interpretation must be evaluated at the population level, for example, as tested sample size increases so does the risk of a detection being a false-positive result. Also, due to the analytical sensitivity of the test, most rtPCR assays classify animals with Ct values greater than 36 to 37 as suspect or inconclusive, as the higher Ct values do not correlate well with gold standard fecal culture results. This is especially true in MAP-infected herds where there is commingling with heavy shedding animals, which can increase the likelihood of ingested organisms from the environment or cross-contamination during sampling. This may cause false-positive testing results, especially for those individuals in the high Ct suspect range. The authors typically recommend resampling and retesting individuals that test in the suspect range after their removal from exposure to or commingling with heavy shedders. These individuals could also be cultured for MAP to determine disease status in high value animals. Interpretation of negative or not detected results also depends on the herd-level status (prevalence) and risk status, as the clinical sensitivity of the assay is ~60%, because animals only shed MAP intermittently in the early stages of disease.[104] Generally, MAP diagnostics and testing programs heavily depend on multiple factors and vary greatly on producer goals, production systems, and herd prevalence, see Sébastien Buczinski and colleagues' article, "Interpretation and Analysis of Individual Diagnostic Tests and Performance," in this issue of Veterinary Clinics for additional information.

Anaerobic Infections

Anaerobic infections in ruminants tend to fall into two major categories: enteric and tissue infections with toxin producing members of the genus *Clostridium* and soft tissue infections caused or associated with Gram-negative, nonspore forming organisms, by members of the genera *Fusobacterium, Bacteroides, Dichelobacter, Porphyromonas,* and *Prevotella.*[105,106] The most significant of the Gram-negative pathogens is *Fusobacterium necrophorum*, which is associated with bovine foot rot and liver abscesses, whereas *Dichelobacter nodosus* is associated with ovine foot rot. Classically, anaerobes provided a significant diagnostic challenge, as they are highly susceptible to oxygen and require specialized sampling, transport, handling, and culture and isolation procedures. In addition, identification based on biochemical testing can be challenging, especially to establish species-level identification of veterinary pathogens. However, robust databases of anaerobic pathogens have been developed for MALDI-TOF, which have proven extremely accurate for identification.[107,108] These advances have greatly improved identification of anaerobes, especially the Gram-negative pathogens described above. If infection with one of these pathogens is suspected, please contact your VDL for specific transport, collection, and submission instructions.

Clostridium perfringens is the primary pathogenic species that causes enterotoxic infections in ruminants, which includes enteritis and abomasitis. Several recent clinical reviews of these diseases in ruminants are available.[109,110] *C perfringens* is classified based on the presence or absence of different toxins genes (Type A–Type G), which make identification alone insufficient for diagnosis. This typing scheme has recently been expanded to reflect two new toxin types, F and G.[111] In VDLs, after isolation and identification of *C perfringens*, isolates are usually subjected to a multiplex toxin typing PCR assay to determine the presence or absence of toxin genes.[111] This is important as *C perfringens* can be found in normal, healthy animals, and isolation from fecal samples may not be clinically relevant. Findings should be interpreted in the context of histopathology and other clinical findings, especially for *C perfringens* Type A.

Clostridium is also responsible for numerous histotoxic and neurotoxic diseases. Histotoxic diseases include clostridial myositis (blackleg) caused by *Clostridium chauvoei* and gas gangrene usually caused by *Clostridium septicum* but also *Clostridium novyi, Clostridium sordellii,* and *C perfringens.*[112] Diagnosis and detection of these agents typically involves identification of organisms associated with lesions. In VDLs, this is performed by fluorescent antibody testing of fixed tissues or tissue smears from affected areas or immunohistochemistry staining of tissue sections.[113,114] Culture and identification of these organisms may be helpful, but interpretation is challenging as they may represent postmortem growth. Neurotoxic diseases associated with *Clostridium* include botulism (*C botulinum*) and tetanus (*C tetani*). Diagnosis of neurotoxic *Clostridium* is usually based on clinical findings and exclusion of other causes; however, culture and identification of the pathogens in lesions may be supportive of the diagnosis. In addition, for botulism, PCR testing for toxins is available for use on clinical samples.[112,115] Methods for detection of preformed botulinum toxin using MALDI-TOF have been developed and used on rumen contents; however, these tests may not be as widely available.[116]

Mastitis

Mastitis, defined as inflammation of the mammary gland, is the most common bacterial disease of adult dairy cows. Mastitis also affects prepubertal and gestational dairy heifers, beef cattle, goats, and sheep. Although usually a disease of females, occasional cases of mastitis are seen in male animals. Mastitis is diagnosed based either on overt clinical signs of inflammation, for example, changes in the appearance of the milk, redness, heat, pain and swelling of the mammary gland, and/or signs of systemic illness, or, for subclinical disease, detection of inflammatory cells (somatic cell count [SCC]) in milk. Mastitis is most frequently caused by a bacterial intramammary infection (IMI). Generally speaking, mastitis-causing bacterial pathogens are grouped into categories based on their clinical behavior (clinical vs subclinical) and/or mode of acquisition. With regard to the latter, pathogens have been classically grouped as contagious, those that spread from animal-to-animal usually during the milking process, and environmental, those that are acquired from the animal's environment between milkings. Among the ruminants commonly encountered in clinical practice, the prevalent bacterial pathogens that cause IMI are generally similar with a few exceptions.

The most commonly isolated bacteria from ruminant milk are the staphylococci, with the so-called non-aureus staphylococci (NAS) being most prevalent. Among the NAS, *Staphylococcus chromogenes* tends to predominate.[117] Some of the NAS species tend to be primarily associated with mammary sources, whereas others tend to be associated with extra-mammary sites, for example, the animal's environment.[118] Common contagious pathogens include *Staphylococcus aureus, Streptococcus agalactiae, Mycoplasma* spp, *Corynebacterium bovis*, and *T pyogenes*. Common environmental pathogens include Gram-negative bacteria including fecal coliforms and Gram-positive bacteria including streptococcal and streptococcal-like organisms other than *S agalactiae,* among which *Streptococcus uberis* and *Streptococcus dysgalactiae* are most frequent. Sheep and goats may also get abscesses in their udder caused by *Corynebacterium pseudotuberculosis*, the causative agent of caseous lymphadenitis, and can have alterations in milk SCC associated with small ruminant lentiviruses.[119]

Diagnosis of the etiology of an IMI is performed to select appropriate treatment protocols and/or initiate preventive measures such as milking time hygiene improvements for contagious bacteria or improvements in bedding management for environmental pathogens. Hence, determining broad groups of pathogens present in milk may be sufficient to implement changes in management or initiate treatment. For example, in the case of clinical mastitis, intramammary treatment is usually limited to Gram-positive infections, whereas diagnosis of subclinical IMI during lactation is usually performed to help guide prevention measures rather than guide treatment as subclinical mastitis is not usually treated during lactation. Currently, bacterial culture and PCR are the most commonly used methods to diagnose IMI.

Bacterial culture of milk is relatively simple to perform and inexpensive.[120] Many mastitis pathogens grow under aerobic conditions on blood agar-based media. There are exceptions, such as *Mycoplasma* spp, which usually require specific growth media and conditions. False-negative results can thus occur when the cow has an IMI with a pathogen that does not grow on routine screening media under aerobic conditions. Although most culture techniques are easily performed, consistent and standardized protocols coupled with established definitions for what constitutes an IMI are necessary to establish a diagnosis. Accurate diagnosis begins with aseptic sample collection.[120] Briefly, teats should be clean and dry and scrubbed with 70% isopropyl alcohol before sample collection. Teats are then stripped of a few streams of milk to reduce the potential for streak canal contaminants in the sample before collecting milk in a sterile vial while wearing disposable gloves. Following collection, samples should be chilled or frozen for transportation to the laboratory. In the laboratory, any frozen samples should be thawed before culture. Using aseptic techniques, a known volume of milk is plated onto culture media and incubated under conditions and times suitable for growth of the potential pathogen(s) of interest.[120] Standardized CFU/mL thresholds are used to define an IMI with a particular pathogen as well as define when a sample is considered contaminated.[121] Generally, a sample is considered contaminated when greater than 2 different colony types are identified in any given sample. Sampling handling is as an important factor to consider when interpreting culture results. Although freezing samples for transportation and/or storage can help reduce bacterial overgrowth in the sample, the impact of storage and freezing on culture results can vary. Some organisms do not always survive freezing or storage for extended periods of time; this includes *E coli*, *T pyogenes*, *Nocardia* spp, and *Mycoplasma* spp. On the other hand, long-term storage does not generally affect the viability of Gram-positive cocci and freezing of milk samples can increase the likelihood of detecting some staphylococcal species and *S aureus*.[122]

Although conventional culture methods are still frequently used to diagnose an IMI, molecular techniques have also become commonplace. The two most common molecular techniques used to diagnose IMI are MALDI-TOF and PCR. Although PCR can be used as a culture-independent method to detect DNA from mastitis-causing organisms directly from the milk sample, MALDI-TOF still requires bacterial culture to isolate the organism of interest. Hence, MALDI-TOF, in its current form, is used to identify isolated organisms to the genus and/or species level. In many laboratories, MALDI-TOF has thus largely replaced traditional biochemistry-based phenotypic methods for identifying bacteria. The method has been validated against traditional phenotypic methods and genotypic methods for bacterial identification and has been found to correctly classify genus and species most of the time, whereas misclassification errors can occur with traditional phenotypic speciation methods for some mastitis pathogens, for example, some species of staphylococci.[123,124] One limitation of MALDI-TOF is that the database used to identify the organism based on its mass spectra must contain the organism of interest. Hence, many mastitis laboratories have developed custom libraries of spectra for mastitis pathogens that are used in concert with the manufacturer's library of organisms to make a diagnosis.[123]

The use of commercially available quantitative rtPCR-based tests for detecting bacterial DNA in milk samples has become quite common in some regions of the world. Advantages of PCR-based techniques include faster turnaround time, user-independent identification of bacteria, and ability to identify organisms that are difficult to culture in a timely fashion, for example, *Mycoplasma* spp. Further, commercially available PCR assays can be directly applied to milk samples containing preservatives, allowing storage and shipment at room temperature and obviating the need for chilled or frozen storage and shipping conditions required for samples undergoing conventional culture. Much like CFU/mL thresholds are used to define an IMI with conventional culture, diagnosis of an IMI with rtPCR is based on the Ct-value needed to detect DNA from a suspected pathogen. With commercial PCR-based tests, the manufacturer determines the Ct-value linked to a diagnosis. Also, like the culture methods, detection of DNA from greater than 2 bacterial genera and/or species indicates contamination. Because PCR detects bacterial DNA, it is possible to detect DNA from organisms that are no longer viable and thus no longer causing an infection. One study comparing conventional culture to PCR longitudinally throughout the course of an infection showed that milk samples remain positive by PCR after conventional cultures have become negative, which could lead to overtreatment of cases where the cow has resolved the infection.[125] Another limitation of PCR-based tests is that the commercial test kit must include PCR primers to detect the organism of interest. Hence, false-negative results can occur when the cow has an infection with an organism for which primers are not included in the test kit.

Although not applied in the routine diagnosis of IMI, a number of molecular methods can be applied to strain-type specific organisms to better understand the epidemiology of mastitis pathogen(s) on farms, for example, to understand contagiousness or better understand reservoir(s) of infection. These methods include, among others, WGS, RAPD-PCR, and pulse-field gel electrophoresis. Metagenomic approaches have also been applied in an effort to understand the milk microbiome.[126] Our understanding of the latter is still in its infancy.

A more comprehensive overview of mastitis diagnostics can be found in the November 2018 edition of VCNA, Food Animal Practice.[127]

SUMMARY

Emerging diagnostic approaches such as rtPCR, MALDI-TOF, and gene sequencing have enhanced diagnostic testing for a variety of infectious diseases in ruminants. rtPCR has enhanced sensitivity, reduced testing time, and minimizes the need for culture. However, interpretation of result requires additional considerations. For MALDI-TOF and WGS, isolation of the pathogen in pure culture is still required. Sequence-based approaches applied directly to clinical samples hold promise for diagnostic testing for these pathogens, but advances in technology, reduction in cost, and ease of analysis need to be comparable with existing methods to be practical.

CLINICS CARE POINTS

- Real-time polymerase chain reaction (PCR) has had a tremendous impact on the ability of VDLs to rapidly detect pathogens in diagnostic samples.
- Multiplexed real-time PCR (rtPCR) syndromic panels have the ability to screen for numerous pathogens simultaneously.
- Interpretation of rtPCR results varies by the clinical disease, pathogen, and sample type. Results may not always directly correlate to culture results or clinical disease, especially with opportunistic pathogens in sites with normal flora.
- Genomic sequencing continues to enhance the ability to identify and characterize bacterial pathogens. When combined with additional technologies such as Matrix -assisted laser desorption ionization–time of flight (MALDI-TOF) and rtPCR, genomic information can be rapidly translated into diagnostic results.

- MALDI-TOF has revolutionized veterinary microbiology and has provided a rapid means to identify most pathogenic bacteria.
- New applications of MALDI-TOF hold promise for strain typing, rapid AMR detection, and use directly on clinical samples.
- Classic culture-based approaches for pathogen isolation continue to be vitally important for bacterial diagnostics, which enable reflex testing like antimicrobial susceptibility, MALDI-TOF typing, and whole -genome sequencing.

STATEMENT

The use of product and company names is necessary to accurately report the methods and results; however, the US Department of Agriculture (USDA) neither guarantees nor warrants the standard of the products, and the use of names by the USDA implies no approval of the product to the exclusion of others that may also be suitable. The USDA is an equal opportunity employer.

DISCLOSURE

Dr. Clawson is supported by USDA/ARS Project # 3040-32000-036-00-D. Dr. Loy is supported by the Nebraska Experiment Station with funds from the Animal Health and Disease Research (section 1433) capacity funding program (Accession 1017646)

REFERENCES

1. Mullis K, Faloona F, Scharf S, et al. Specific enzymatic amplification of DNA in vitro: the polymerase chain reaction. Cold Spring Harbor Symposia Quantitative Biol 1986;51:263–73.
2. Toohey-Kurth KL, Mulrooney DM, Hinkley S, et al. Best practices for performance of real-time PCR assays in veterinary diagnostic laboratories. J Vet Diagn Invest 2020;32(6):815–25.
3. Bustin SA, Benes V, Garson JA, et al. The MIQE guidelines: minimum information for publication of quantitative real-time PCR experiments. Clin Chem 2009;55(4):611–22.
4. Gunson RN, Bennett S, Maclean A, et al. Using multiplex real time PCR in order to streamline a routine diagnostic service. J Clin Virol 2008;43(4):372–5.
5. Loy JD, Leger L, Workman AM, et al. Development of a multiplex real-time PCR assay using two thermocycling platforms for detection of major bacterial pathogens associated with bovine respiratory disease complex from clinical samples. J Vet Diagn Invest 2018;30(6):837–47.
6. Hoffmann B, Depner K, Schirrmeier H, et al. A universal heterologous internal control system for duplex real-time RT-PCR assays used in a detection system for pestiviruses. J Virol Methods 2006;136(1–2):200–9.
7. Randall LP, Lemma F, Koylass M, et al. Evaluation of MALDI-ToF as a method for the identification of bacteria in the veterinary diagnostic laboratory. Res Vet Sci 2015;101:42–9.
8. Wragg P, Randall L, Whatmore AM. Comparison of Biolog GEN III MicroStation semi-automated bacterial identification system with matrix-assisted laser desorption ionization-time of flight mass spectrometry and 16S ribosomal RNA gene sequencing for the identification of bacteria of veterinary interest. J Microbiol Methods 2014;105:16–21.

9. Khot PD, Couturier MR, Wilson A, et al. Optimization of matrix-assisted laser desorption ionization–time of flight mass spectrometry analysis for bacterial identification. J Clin Microbiol 2012;50(12):3845–52.
10. Wilson David J, Middleton John R, Adkins Pamela RF, et al. Test agreement among biochemical methods, matrix-assisted laser desorption ionization–time of flight mass spectrometry, and 16S rRNA sequencing for identification of microorganisms isolated from bovine milk. J Clin Microbiol 2019;57(3):013811-18.
11. Robbins K, Dickey AM, Clawson ML, et al. Matrix-assisted laser desorption/ionization time-of-flight mass spectrometry identification of Moraxella bovoculi and Moraxella bovis isolates from cattle. J Vet Diagn Invest 2018;30(5):739–42.
12. Kuhnert P, Bisgaard M, Korczak BM, et al. Identification of animal Pasteurellaceae by MALDI-TOF mass spectrometry. J Microbiol Methods 2012;89(1):1–7.
13. Spergser J, Hess C, Loncaric I, et al. Matrix-Assisted laser desorption ionization–time of flight mass spectrometry is a superior diagnostic tool for the identification and differentiation of mycoplasmas isolated from animals. J Clin Microbiol 2019;57(9):e00316-9.
14. Loy JD, Clawson ML. Rapid typing of Mannheimia haemolytica major genotypes 1 and 2 using MALDI-TOF mass spectrometry. J Microbiol Methods 2017; 136:30–3.
15. Hille M, Dickey A, Robbins K, et al. Rapid differentiation of Moraxella bovoculi genotypes 1 and 2 using MALDI-TOF mass spectrometry profiles. J Microbiol Methods 2020;173:105942.
16. Mani RJ, Thachil AJ, Ramachandran A. Discrimination of Streptococcus equi subsp. equi and Streptococcus equi subsp. zooepidemicus using matrix-assisted laser desorption/ionization time-of-flight mass spectrometry. J Vet Diagn Invest 2017;29(5):622–7.
17. Berrazeg M, Diene SM, Drissi M, et al. Biotyping of Multidrug-Resistant Klebsiella pneumoniae Clinical Isolates from France and Algeria Using MALDI-TOF MS. PLoS One 2013;8(4):e61428.
18. Bobay LM, Ochman H. The evolution of bacterial genome architecture. Front Genet 2017;8:72.
19. Pfeifer E, de Sousa JAM, Touchon M, et al. Bacteria have numerous distinctive groups of phage-plasmids with conserved phage and variable plasmid gene repertoires. Nucleic Acids Res 2021;49(5):2655–73.
20. Andreani NA, Hesse E, Vos M. Prokaryote genome fluidity is dependent on effective population size. ISME J 2017;11(7):1719–21.
21. Partridge SR, Kwong SM, Firth N, et al. Mobile genetic elements associated with antimicrobial resistance. Clin Microbiol Rev 2018;31(4). https://doi.org/10.1128/CMR.00088-17.
22. Siguier P, Gourbeyre E, Chandler M. Bacterial insertion sequences: their genomic impact and diversity. FEMS Microbiol Rev 2014;38(5):865–91.
23. Mazel D. Integrons: agents of bacterial evolution. Nat Rev Microbiol 2006;4(8): 608–20.
24. Zhou K, Aertsen A, Michiels CW. The role of variable DNA tandem repeats in bacterial adaptation. FEMS Microbiol Rev 2014;38(1):119–41.
25. Chen J, Leblanc DJ, Galli DM. DNA inversion on conjugative plasmid pVT745. J Bacteriol 2002;184(21):5926–34.
26. Merrikh CN, Merrikh H. Gene inversion potentiates bacterial evolvability and virulence. Nat Commun 2018;9(1):4662.
27. Ramiro RS, Durao P, Bank C, et al. Low mutational load and high mutation rate variation in gut commensal bacteria. Plos Biol 2020;18(3):e3000617.

28. Weinroth MD, Clawson ML, Arthur TM, et al. Rates of evolutionary change of resident Escherichia coli O157:H7 differ within the same ecological niche. BMC Genomics 2022;23(1):275.
29. Ehrlich GD, Hiller NL, Hu FZ. What makes pathogens pathogenic. Genome Biol 2008;9(6):225.
30. Hu T, Chitnis N, Monos D, et al. Next-generation sequencing technologies: an overview. Hum Immunol 2021. https://doi.org/10.1016/j.humimm.2021.02.012.
31. Slatko BE, Gardner AF, Ausubel FM. Overview of Next-Generation Sequencing Technologies. Curr Protoc Mol Biol 2018;122(1):e59.
32. Phillippy AM, Schatz MC, Pop M. Genome assembly forensics: finding the elusive mis-assembly. Genome Biol 2008;9(3):R55.
33. Koren S, Harhay GP, Smith TP, et al. Reducing assembly complexity of microbial genomes with single-molecule sequencing. Genome Biol 2013;14(9):R101.
34. Clawson ML, Schuller G, Dickey AM, et al. Differences between predicted outer membrane proteins of genotype 1 and 2 Mannheimia haemolytica. BMC Microbiol 2020;20(1):250.
35. Bickhart DM, Kolmogorov M, Tseng E, et al. Generating lineage-resolved, complete metagenome-assembled genomes from complex microbial communities. Nat Biotechnol 2022. https://doi.org/10.1038/s41587-021-01130-z.
36. Franco-Duarte R, Cernakova L, Kadam S, et al. Advances in chemical and biological methods to identify microorganisms-from past to present. Microorganisms 2019;7(5). https://doi.org/10.3390/microorganisms7050130.
37. Kamble A, Sawant S, Singh H. 16S ribosomal RNA gene-based metagenomics: a review. Biomed Res J 2020;7:5–11.
38. Yang B, Wang Y, Qian PY. Sensitivity and correlation of hypervariable regions in 16S rRNA genes in phylogenetic analysis. BMC Bioinformatics 2016;17:135.
39. Glaeser SP, Kampfer P. Multilocus sequence analysis (MLSA) in prokaryotic taxonomy. Syst Appl Microbiol 2015;38(4):237–45.
40. Sant'Anna FH, Bach E, Porto RZ, et al. Genomic metrics made easy: what to do and where to go in the new era of bacterial taxonomy. Crit Rev Microbiol 2019; 45(2):182–200.
41. Yoon SH, Ha SM, Lim J, et al. A large-scale evaluation of algorithms to calculate average nucleotide identity. Antonie Van Leeuwenhoek 2017;110(10):1281–6.
42. Parks DH, Chuvochina M, Chaumeil PA, et al. A complete domain-to-species taxonomy for Bacteria and Archaea. Nat Biotechnol 2020;38(9):1079–86.
43. Richter M, Rossello-Mora R, Oliver Glockner F, et al. JSpeciesWS: a web server for prokaryotic species circumscription based on pairwise genome comparison. Bioinformatics 2016;32(6):929–31.
44. Ciufo S, Kannan S, Sharma S, et al. Using average nucleotide identity to improve taxonomic assignments in prokaryotic genomes at the NCBI. Int J Syst Evol Microbiol 2018;68(7):2386–92.
45. Dickey AM, Loy JD, Bono JL, et al. Large genomic differences between Moraxella bovoculi isolates acquired from the eyes of cattle with infectious bovine keratoconjunctivitis versus the deep nasopharynx of asymptomatic cattle. Vet Res 2016;47:31.
46. Wynn EL, Hille MM, Loy JD, et al. Whole genome sequencing of diverse Moraxella bovis strains reveals two genotypes with different genetic determinants. BMC Microbiol 2022;22:258. https://doi.org/10.1186/s12866-022-02670-3.
47. Griffin D, Chengappa MM, Kuszak J, et al. Bacterial pathogens of the bovine respiratory disease complex. Vet Clin North Am Food Anim Pract 2010;26(2): 381–94.

48. Goecke NB, Nielsen BH, Petersen MB, et al. Design of a high-throughput real-time PCR system for detection of bovine respiratory and enteric pathogens. original research. Front Vet Sci 2021. https://doi.org/10.3389/fvets.2021.677993.

49. Pansri P, Katholm J, Krogh KM, et al. Evaluation of novel multiplex qPCR assays for diagnosis of pathogens associated with the bovine respiratory disease complex. Vet J 2020;256:105425.

50. Wisselink HJ, Cornelissen JBWJ, van der Wal FJ, et al. Evaluation of a multiplex real-time PCR for detection of four bacterial agents commonly associated with bovine respiratory disease in bronchoalveolar lavage fluid. BMC Vet Res 2017;13(1):221.

51. Goto Y, Yaegashi G, Fukunari K, et al. Design of a multiplex quantitative reverse transcription-PCR system to simultaneously detect 16 pathogens associated with bovine respiratory and enteric diseases. J Appl Microbiol 2020;129(4):832–47.

52. Horwood PF, Mahony TJ. Multiplex real-time RT-PCR detection of three viruses associated with the bovine respiratory disease complex. J Virol Methods 2011;171(2):360–3.

53. Buczinski S, Pardon B. Bovine respiratory disease diagnosis: what progress has been made in clinical diagnosis? Vet Clin North Am Food Anim Pract 2020;36(2):399–423.

54. Bell CJ, Blackburn P, Elliott M, et al. Investigation of polymerase chain reaction assays to improve detection of bacterial involvement in bovine respiratory disease. J Vet Diagn Invest 2014;26(5):631–4.

55. Sachse K, Salam HSH, Diller R, et al. Use of a novel real-time PCR technique to monitor and quantitate Mycoplasma bovis infection in cattle herds with mastitis and respiratory disease. Vet J 2010;186(3):299–303.

56. Fulton RW, Confer AW. Laboratory test descriptions for bovine respiratory disease diagnosis and their strengths and weaknesses: gold standards for diagnosis, do they exist? Can Vet J 2012;53(7):754–61.

57. Klompmaker AF, Brydensholt M, Michelsen AM, et al. Estimating clinically relevant cut-off values for a high-throughput quantitative real-time PCR detecting bacterial respiratory pathogens in cattle. Brief research report. Front Vet Sci 2021;8:674771. https://doi.org/10.3389/fvets.2021.674771.

58. Workman AM, Kuehn LA, McDaneld TG, et al. Longitudinal study of humoral immunity to bovine coronavirus, virus shedding, and treatment for bovine respiratory disease in pre-weaned beef calves. BMC Vet Res 2019;15(1):161.

59. Workman AM, Kuehn LA, McDaneld TG, et al. Evaluation of the effect of serum antibody abundance against bovine coronavirus on bovine coronavirus shedding and risk of respiratory tract disease in beef calves from birth through the first five weeks in a feedlot. Am J Vet Res 2017;78(9):1065–76.

60. Dutta E, Loy JD, Deal CA, et al. Development of a multiplex real-time PCR assay for predicting macrolide and tetracycline resistance associated with bacterial pathogens of bovine respiratory disease. Pathogens 2021;10(1). https://doi.org/10.3390/pathogens10010064.

61. Freeman CN, Herman EK, Abi Younes J, et al. Evaluating the potential of third generation metagenomic sequencing for the detection of BRD pathogens and genetic determinants of antimicrobial resistance in chronically ill feedlot cattle. BMC Vet Res 2022;18(1):211.

62. Clawson ML, Murray RW, Sweeney MT, et al. Genomic signatures of Mannheimia haemolytica that associate with the lungs of cattle with respiratory disease, an

integrative conjugative element, and antibiotic resistance genes. BMC Genomics 2016;17(1):982.

63. Van Driessche L, Bokma J, Deprez P, et al. Rapid identification of respiratory bacterial pathogens from bronchoalveolar lavage fluid in cattle by MALDI-TOF MS. Scientific Rep 2019;9(1):18381.

64. Van Driessche L, Bokma J, Gille L, et al. Rapid detection of tetracycline resistance in bovine Pasteurella multocida isolates by MALDI Biotyper antibiotic susceptibility test rapid assay (MBT-ASTRA). Scientific Rep 2018;8(1). https://doi.org/10.1038/s41598-018-31562-8.

65. Martin MS, Grau SA, Rutherford BW, et al. Survey of cow-calf producer perspectives on management strategies and industry challenges. Part 1: handling practices, and health and industry challenges. Translational Anim Sci 2018;3(1):195–203.

66. Loy JD, Hille M, Maier G, et al. Component causes of infectious bovine keratoconjunctivitis - the role of moraxella species in the epidemiology of infectious bovine keratoconjunctivitis. Vet Clin North Am Food Anim Pract 2021/07/01/2021;37(2):279–93.

67. Loy JD, Clothier KA, Maier G. Component causes of infectious bovine keratoconjunctivitis—non-moraxella organisms in the epidemiology of infectious bovine keratoconjunctivitis. Vet Clin North Am Food Anim Pract 2021;37(2):295–308.

68. Zheng W, Porter E, Noll L, et al. A multiplex real-time PCR assay for the detection and differentiation of five bovine pinkeye pathogens. J Microbiol Methods 2019;160:87–92.

69. Schmellik-Sandage CS, Hill RE Jr. Regulation of autogenous biologicals in the United States. Dev biologicals 2004;117:9–13.

70. Rogers DG, Cheville NF, Pugh GW Jr. Pathogenesis of corneal lesions caused by Moraxella bovis in gnotobiotic calves. Vet Pathol 1987;24(4):287–95.

71. Loy JD, Brodersen BW. Moraxella spp. isolated from field outbreaks of infectious bovine keratoconjunctivitis: a retrospective study of case submissions from 2010 to 2013. J Vet Diagn Invest 2014;26(6):761–8.

72. Hille MM, Clawson ML, Dickey AM, et al. MALDI-TOF MS Biomarker Detection Models to Distinguish RTX toxin phenotypes of moraxella bovoculi strains are enhanced using calcium chloride supplemented agar. Original Research. Front Cell Infect Microbiol 2021;11(202). https://doi.org/10.3389/fcimb.2021.632647.

73. Mee JF. Investigation of bovine abortion and stillbirth/perinatal mortality - similar diagnostic challenges, different approaches. Irish Vet J 2020;73(1). https://doi.org/10.1186/s13620-020-00172-0.

74. Clothier K, Anderson M. Evaluation of bovine abortion cases and tissue suitability for identification of infectious agents in California diagnostic laboratory cases from 2007 to 2012. Theriogenology 2016;85(5):933–8.

75. Kirkbride CA. Bacterial agents detected in a lo-year study of bovine abortions and stillbirths. J Vet Diagn Invest 1993;5(1):64–8.

76. Wolf-Jäckel GA, Strube ML, Schou KK, et al. Bovine Abortions Revisited—Enhancing Abortion Diagnostics by 16S rDNA Amplicon Sequencing and Fluorescence in situ Hybridization. Original Research. Front Vet Sci 2021. https://doi.org/10.3389/fvets.2021.623666.

77. Cabell E. Bovine abortion: aetiology and investigations. Practice 2007;29(8):455–63.

78. Botta C, Pellegrini G, Hässig M, et al. Bovine fetal placenta during pregnancy and the postpartum period. Vet Pathol 2018;56(2):248–58.

79. Tramuta C, Lacerenza D, Zoppi S, et al. Development of a set of multiplex standard polymerase chain reaction assays for the identification of infectious agents from aborted bovine clinical samples. J Vet Diagn Invest 2011;23(4):657–64.
80. Brooks RS, Blanchard MT, Clothier KA, et al. Characterization of Pajaroellobacter abortibovis, the etiologic agent of epizootic bovine abortion. Vet Microbiol 2016;192:73–80.
81. Pereira GR, Vogel FSF, Bohrer RC, et al. Neospora caninum DNA detection by TaqMan real-time PCR assay in experimentally infected pregnant heifers. Vet Parasitol 2014;199(3):129–35.
82. Stoddard RA, Gee JE, Wilkins PP, et al. Detection of pathogenic Leptospira spp. through TaqMan polymerase chain reaction targeting the LipL32 gene. Diagn Microbiol Infect Dis 2009;64(3):247–55.
83. Mahlum CE, Haugerud S, Shivers JL, et al. Detection of bovine viral diarrhea virus by TaqMan® reverse transcription polymerase chain reaction. J Vet Diagn Invest 2002;14(2):120–5.
84. McAllister MM. Diagnosis and control of bovine neosporosis. Vet Clin North Am Food Anim Pract 2016/07/01/2016;32(2):443–63.
85. Whitman KJ, Bono JL, Clawson ML, et al. Genomic-based identification of environmental and clinical Listeria monocytogenes strains associated with an abortion outbreak in beef heifers. BMC Vet Res 2020;16(1):70.
86. Foster DM, Smith GW. Pathophysiology of diarrhea in calves. Vet Clin North Am Food Anim Pract 2009;25(1):13–36.
87. Blanchard PC. Diagnostics of dairy and beef cattle diarrhea. Vet Clin North Am Food Anim Pract 2012;28(3):443–64.
88. Cho Y-I, Kim W-I, Liu S, et al. Development of a panel of multiplex real-time polymerase chain reaction assays for simultaneous detection of major agents causing calf diarrhea in feces. J Vet Diagn Invest 2010;22(4):509–17.
89. Cho Y-I, Sun D, Cooper V, et al. Evaluation of a commercial rapid test kit for detecting bovine enteric pathogens in feces. J Vet Diagn Invest 2012;24(3):559–62.
90. Heller MC, Chigerwe M. Diagnosis and treatment of infectious enteritis in neonatal and juvenile ruminants. Vet Clin North Am Food Anim Pract 2018;34(1):101–17.
91. Gyles CL, Fairbrother JM. Escherichia coli. Pathogenesis Bacterial Infections Anim 2010;267–308. https://doi.org/10.1002/9780470958209.ch15. Wiley Online Books.
92. Moxley RA, Smith DR. Attaching-effacing escherichia coli infections in cattle. Vet Clin North Am Food Anim Pract 2010;26(1):29–56.
93. Franck SM, Bosworth BT, Moon HW. Multiplex PCR for Enterotoxigenic, Attaching and Effacing, and Shiga Toxin-Producing Escherichia coli Strains from Calves. J Clin Microbiol 1998;36(6):1795–7.
94. Barrow PA, Jones MA, Thomson N. Salmonella. Pathogenesis Bacterial Infections Anim 2010;231–65. https://doi.org/10.1002/9780470958209.ch14. Wiley Online Books.
95. Gutema FD, Agga GE, Abdi RD, et al. Prevalence and serotype diversity of salmonella in apparently healthy cattle: systematic review and meta-analysis of published studies, 2000–2017. Systematic Review. Front Vet Sci 2019;6:102. https://doi.org/10.3389/fvets.2019.00102.
96. Nielsen LR. Review of pathogenesis and diagnostic methods of immediate relevance for epidemiology and control of Salmonella Dublin in cattle. Vet Microbiol 2013;162(1):1–9.

97. Goodman LB, McDonough PL, Anderson RR, et al. Detection of Salmonella spp. in veterinary samples by combining selective enrichment and real-time PCR. J Vet Diagn Invest 2017;29(6):844–51.

98. Nielsen LR, Ersbøll AK. Age-stratified validation of an indirect salmonella dublin serum enzyme-linked immunosorbent assay for individual diagnosis in cattle. J Vet Diagn Invest 2004;16(3):212–8.

99. Mohler VL, Izzo MM, House JK. Salmonella in calves. Vet Clin North Am Food Anim Pract 2009;25(1):37–54.

100. Holschbach CL, Peek SF. Salmonella in dairy cattle. Vet Clin North Am Food Anim Pract 2018;34(1):133–54.

101. Collins MT. Diagnosis of paratuberculosis. Vet Clin North Am Food Anim Pract 2011;27(3):581–91.

102. Grant IR. Bacteriophage-Based Methods for Detection of Viable Mycobacterium avium subsp. paratuberculosis and Their Potential for Diagnosis of Johne's Disease. Mini Review. Front Vet Sci 2021;8:632498. https://doi.org/10.3389/fvets.2021.632498.

103. Collins MT, Gardner IA, Garry FB, et al. Consensus recommendations on diagnostic testing for the detection of paratuberculosis in cattle in the United States. J Am Vet Med Assoc 2006;229(12):1912–9.

104. Alinovi CA, Ward MP, Lin TL, et al. Real-time PCR, compared to liquid and solid culture media and ELISA, for the detection of Mycobacterium avium ssp. paratuberculosis. Vet Microbiol 2009;136(1–2):177–9.

105. Nagaraja TG. Gram-negative, non-spore-forming anaerobes. Vet Microbiol 2022;294–308.

106. Gohari IM, Prescott JF. Clostridium. Vet Microbiol 2022;309–34.

107. Alcalá L, Marín M, Ruiz A, et al. Identifying Anaerobic Bacteria Using MALDI-TOF mass spectrometry: a four-year experience. Original Research. Front Cell Infect Microbiol 2021;11:521014. https://doi.org/10.3389/fcimb.2021.521014.

108. Justesen Ulrik S, Holm A, Knudsen E, et al. Species identification of clinical isolates of anaerobic bacteria: a comparison of two matrix-assisted laser desorption ionization–time of flight mass spectrometry systems. J Clin Microbiol 2011;49(12):4314–8.

109. Simpson KM, Callan RJ, Van Metre DC. Clostridial abomasitis and enteritis in ruminants. Vet Clin North Am Food Anim Pract 2018;34(1):155–84.

110. Otter A, Uzal FA. Clostridial diseases in farm animals: 1. Enterotoxaemias and other alimentary tract infections. Practice 2020;42(4):219–32. https://doi.org/10.1136/inp.m1462.

111. Rood JI, Adams V, Lacey J, et al. Expansion of the Clostridium perfringens toxin-based typing scheme. Anaerobe 2018;53:5–10.

112. Otter A, Uzal FA. Clostridial diseases in farm animals: 2. Histotoxic and neurotoxic diseases. Practice 2020;42(5):279–88, m1984.

113. Uzal FA, Paramidani M, Assis R, et al. Outbreak of clostridial myocarditis in calves. Vet Rec 2003;152(5):134–6.

114. Sterne M, Batty I. Pathogenic clostridia. London WC2B 6AB.: Butterworth & Co.(Publishers) Ltd, 88 Kingsway; 1975.

115. De Medici D, Anniballi F, Wyatt Gary M, et al. Multiplex PCR for Detection of Botulinum Neurotoxin-Producing Clostridia in Clinical, Food, and Environmental Samples. Appl Environ Microbiol 2009;75(20):6457–61.

116. Frye EA, Egan C, Perry MJ, et al. Outbreak of botulism type A in dairy cows detected by MALDI-TOF mass spectrometry. J Vet Diagn Invest 2020;32(5):722–6.

117. Fry PR, Middleton JR, Dufour S, et al. Association of coagulase-negative staphylococcal species, mammary quarter milk somatic cell count, and persistence of intramammary infection in dairy cattle. J Dairy Sci 2014;97(8):4876–85.

118. De Visscher A, Supre K, Haesebrouck F, et al. Further evidence for the existence of environmental and host-associated species of coagulase-negative staphylococci in dairy cattle. Vet Microbiol 2014;172(3–4):466–74.

119. Sanchez A, Contreras A, Corrales JC, et al. Relationships between infection with caprine arthritis encephalitis virus, intramammary bacterial infection and somatic cell counts in dairy goats. Vet Rec 2001;148(23):711–4.

120. Middleton JR, Fox LK, Pighetti G, et al. Laboratory Handbook on Bovine Mastitis. 3rd. New Prague: National Mastitis Council; 2017.

121. Dohoo IR, Smith J, Andersen S, et al. Diagnosing intramammary infections: evaluation of definitions based on a single milk sample. J Dairy Sci 2011;94(1):250–61.

122. Schukken YH, Grommers FJ, Smit JA, et al. Effect of freezing on bacteriologic culturing of mastitis milk samples. J Dairy Sci 1989;72(7):1900–6.

123. Cameron M, Perry J, Middleton JR, et al. Short communication: Evaluation of MALDI-TOF mass spectrometry and a custom reference spectra expanded database for the identification of bovine-associated coagulase-negative staphylococci. J Dairy Sci 2018;101(1):590–5.

124. Park JY, Fox LK, Seo KS, et al. Comparison of phenotypic and genotypic methods for the species identification of coagulase-negative staphylococcal isolates from bovine intramammary infections. Vet Microbiol 2011;147(1–2):142–8.

125. Hiitio H, Pyorala S, Taponen S, et al. Elimination of experimentally induced bovine intramammary infection assessed by multiplex real-time PCR and bacterial culture. J Dairy Sci 2018;101(6):5267–76.

126. Ruegg PL. The bovine milk microbiome - an evolving science. Domest Anim Endocrinol 2022;79:106708.

127. Adkins PRF, Middleton JR. Methods for diagnosing mastitis. Vet Clin North Am Food Anim Pract 2018;34(3):479–91.

Application and Interpretation of Antimicrobial Susceptibility Testing

Virginia R. Fajt, DVM, PhD[a],*, Brian V. Lubbers, DVM, PhD[b]

KEYWORDS

- Antimicrobial susceptibility testing • Breakpoints • Bacterial infections
- Diagnostic laboratory • Pharmacokinetics
- Pharmacokinetic-pharmacodynamic integration

KEY POINTS

- Antimicrobial susceptibility testing (AST) can provide case-specific information about the likelihood of clinical outcome for bacterial isolates from cattle with cattle-specific breakpoints.

- AST may provide case-specific information about the likelihood of clinical outcome when there are no approved breakpoints for the specific bacterial species and antimicrobial drug. Breakpoints approved for other species of animals should be applied cautiously. Additional sources of information can be consulted for more specific recommendations.

- Absence of breakpoints for a particular drug-bacterial species combination does not necessarily indicate lack of clinical effectiveness. There are a number of reasons why breakpoints have not been approved for some drugs.

- There are no approved breakpoints in any species of animal for bacteria isolated from the gastrointestinal tract that predict clinical outcome of enteric disease. Results from gentamicin and neomycin AST have not been demonstrated to predict outcomes for enteric isolates.

- Breakpoints are tied to a particular antimicrobial regimen. If a different regimen or formulation is being used, the breakpoints may or may not apply.

- Breakpoints are only approved for injectable and intramammary antimicrobials and do not apply to antimicrobials administered in the feed or water such as chlortetracycline, oxytetracycline, tylosin, and sulfonamides because of pharmacokinetic difference.

[a] Veterinary Physiology and Pharmacology, Texas A&M University, 4466 TAMU, College Station, TX 77843, USA; [b] Food Animal Therapeutics - Outreach, Kansas State University, P203 Mosier Hall, Manhattan, KS 66506, USA
* Corresponding author.
E-mail address: vfajt@tamu.edu

Vet Clin Food Anim 39 (2023) 115–128
https://doi.org/10.1016/j.cvfa.2022.09.001

INTRODUCTION

More than 70 years ago, 5 isolates of bacteria from calves with diarrhea were declared "resistant" to antibiotics.[1] On critical review of the results, however, this resistance seems to be based on an arbitrary assessment of the minimal inhibitory concentration. This report demonstrates a sharp contrast to the methods used in modern bacteriology and diagnostic laboratories, which typically use standardized methods for isolating and identifying bacteria and standardized criteria for categorizing bacterial isolates as susceptible or resistant. Where do those standards come from, and are they accurate for bacterial isolates from cattle? Moreover, how do those standards affect veterinarians' interpretation of antimicrobial susceptibility data?

In this article, we will describe how antimicrobial susceptibility testing (AST) is an important part of antimicrobial stewardship, how the test methods and interpretive criteria for AST are developed, when AST might or might not be useful in clinical practice, and how to interpret AST data from individual cases, antibiograms, and published literature. We will not address AST or antimicrobial resistance in the context of food safety or human health risk, such as the interpretation of AST from commensal *Escherichia coli* or other bacteria that are nonpathogenic to ruminants and are assessed as part of antimicrobial resistance surveillance programs such as the National Antimicrobial Resistance Monitoring System for Enteric Bacteria. Instead, we will focus on AST that informs animal health and antimicrobial decision-making in veterinary medicine.

ANTIMICROBIAL SUSCEPTIBILITY TESTING AND ANTIMICROBIAL STEWARDSHIP

As defined by the American Veterinary Medical Association (AVMA), antimicrobial stewardship refers to "the actions veterinarians take individually and as a profession to preserve the effectiveness and availability of antimicrobial drugs through conscientious oversight and responsible medical decision-making while safeguarding animal, public, and environmental health."[2] This aligns with the definition from the American Association of Bovine Practitioners, which is "Commitment to reducing the need for antimicrobial drugs by preventing infectious disease in cattle, and when antimicrobial drugs are needed, to using antimicrobial drugs appropriately to optimize health outcomes and minimize selection for antimicrobial resistance as well as prevent violative residues."[3] The American Association of Small Ruminant Practitioners also promotes antimicrobial stewardship and endorses the AVMA definition.[4] An important function of antimicrobial stewardship is making evidence-based decisions about which antimicrobials to use. Evidence-based in this context means choosing antimicrobials that are likely to be effective, and compelling evidence of effectiveness can come from several sources:

1. high-quality controlled clinical trials that are published in the peer-reviewed literature or studies conducted as part of a drug label approval,
2. high-quality controlled clinical trials that are conducted internally on large cattle or small ruminant operations,
3. observational studies with appropriate controls for confounding and bias such as selection and allocation bias, and
4. in vitro AST results that are performed under standardized conditions, using interpretive criteria that have are based on clinical studies in cattle or validated pharmacokinetic-pharmacodynamic integration and modeling.

This does not suggest that sources (1) and (2) are more or less important but they also usually represent a small cross-section of cattle production systems, they may not be representative of the disease seen in a specific clinical scenario, and they may be so tightly controlled as to poorly represent everyday animal production practices or veterinary medical practices. AST on isolates from the affected animals provides data that are relevant in space and time. However, in order to provide compelling evidence of effectiveness, AST must be performed appropriately and the results interpreted correctly, as we describe in the next sections.

HOW AST IS PERFORMED AND HOW AST STANDARDS AND BREAKPOINTS ARE DEVELOPED

The essential diagnostic purpose of AST is to use in vitro data, that is, the concentration of an antimicrobial needed to inhibit the growth of a clinical bacterial isolate, to predict a clinical disease outcome in an animal. The minimal inhibitory concentrations (MICs) or zone diameters used to categorize a bacterial isolate as "susceptible" or "resistant" are called breakpoints. In well-designed AST, the concentrations measured in the laboratory in vitro correlate with achievable concentrations of antimicrobials in the animal *and* there is evidence that animals clinically affected with bacteria with MICs in the "susceptible" range are likely to respond to treatment. AST identifies the *phenotype* of the bacterial isolate, that is, the quantification of how much drug is needed to inhibit growth, by interpreting the MIC or zone diameter using established breakpoints. This differs from a resistance *genotype*, which indicates the presence of a gene that confers resistance. An important note: There are published articles that show that different media (eg, media supplemented with bovine serum) can result in a different AST result for a bacterial isolate. These reports suggest that efforts to more precisely mimic in vivo conditions, by altering the test media used in vitro, for example, are superior, which misses the point of standardized AST testing. The objective is not to mimic in vivo conditions but rather the goal is to develop a highly standardized, repeatable test that correlates to clinical outcome.

A perfect clinical study of a fictitious antimicrobial, Purplemycin, that demonstrates correlation between MICs in vitro to clinical cure in vivo might look like this: 300 animals developed naturally occurring respiratory disease, bacteria culture was performed from bronchoalveolar lavage samples collected before treatment, broth microdilution AST was performed, animals were treated with Purplemycin (5 mg/kg SC once), and clinical outcome was recorded as shown in **Table 1**. All other things being equal, these data suggest that the breakpoint for susceptibility for this drug and this species of bacteria would be 0.25 µg/mL or lesser, and that the breakpoint for resistance would be greater than 0.5 µg/mL.

In reality, MIC data are not usually 100% correlated to clinical outcome, especially for multifactorial diseases such as bovine respiratory disease, and additional data are

Table 1	
Clinical outcomes of a hypothetical clinical trial based on MICs of bacterial isolates	
MIC (Number of Isolates)	**Clinical Outcome**
0.06 µg/mL (50)	No retreatment required
0.12 µg/mL (50)	No retreatment required
0.25 µg/mL (50)	No retreatment required
1 µg/mL (50)	Died
2 µg/mL (50)	Died
4 µg/mL (50)	Died

Table 2
PK/PD targets for antimicrobial drugs

Category	PK/PD Parameter	PK/PD in Words[a]	Antimicrobial Groups
Time-dependent	$f\%T > MIC$	Percent of time that unbound drug stays above the MIC of the isolate	β-lactams Cephalosporins Carbapenems
Concentration-dependent	$fAUC{:}MIC$	Ratio of area under the time-concentration curve of unbound drug (>24-h period) to the MIC of the isolate	Fluoroquinolones Tetracyclines Maybe sulfonamides Maybe macrolides Maybe phenicols
Concentration-dependent	$fC_{max}{:}MIC$	Ratio of peak concentration of unbound drug to the MIC of the isolate	Aminoglycosides MAYBE fluoroquinolones

[a] See CLSI VET02 for details on targets.[5]

required by standards setting bodies to set these breakpoints. The Clinical and Laboratory Standards Institute (CLSI) is the standard setting body that approves the breakpoints used by most diagnostic laboratories in North America. For example, it would be more convincing if we also had pharmacokinetic data that supported the dosing regimen and demonstrated that the concentrations of the drug are likely to correlate with the concentrations that seems to have the desired clinical effect (pharmacokinetic-pharmacodynamic integration or PK/PD; **Table 2** for PK/PD targets by antimicrobial drug group). However, this illustrates one of the core components of breakpoint development: MIC versus the clinical outcome expected when antimicrobial drugs are used, such as "no retreatment required" in the example above. In some circumstance, clinical outcomes may not be required to be completed at the same time as the PK and PK/PD data collection and analysis. The details and mathematical/statistical approaches to developing breakpoints from PK and PK/PD are beyond the scope of this article and are outlined in detail in other resources.[5–9] However, the commonly used sources of data for developing breakpoints are illustrated in **Fig. 1**.

DECIDING WHEN TO DO ANTIMICROBIAL SUSCEPTIBILITY TESTING

Getting the best results from tests performed by a laboratory includes developing a close working relationship with laboratory personnel. Because the test result is only as good as the sample, diagnostic test results rely on good sample collection with an understanding of how the testing is performed, and laboratory personnel can provide instructions and feedback on sample collection, storage, processing, and shipping. Many diagnostic laboratories have how-to guides or videos, and guidance has also been published.[10]

Decisions about whether to perform AST can be based on the disease or indication (**Table 3**) and on the bacterial species isolated. AST can be useful when the suspected infecting bacterial organism is at risk of acquired resistance, such as bacterial isolates from the families *Pasteurellaceae* or *Enterobacterales*. AST is generally *not* recommended when bacterial isolates are universally susceptible to a drug or drug class (such as beta-hemolytic Streptococci and penicillin), or they are intrinsically resistant

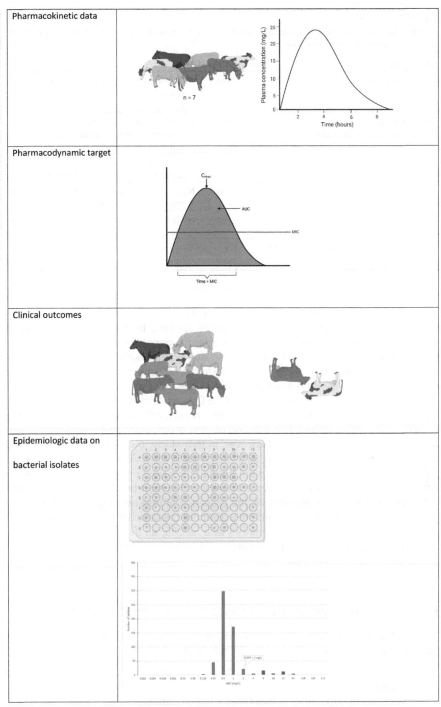

Fig. 1. Data sources for developing breakpoints for antimicrobial drugs to categorize bacterial isolates as susceptible or resistant.

Table 3
Approaches to choosing whether to culture and perform antimicrobial susceptibility testing on bacterial isolates from cattle

Indication	Culture	AST	
Calf/kid/lamb diarrhea	Yes	No	No breakpoints approved for enteric disease because PK/PD targets are unknown
Respiratory disease/bronchopneumonia	Yes	Yes	Consider culturing at necropsy, nonresponders, and for surveillance purposes to monitor trends over time
Mastitis	Yes	+/−	May be valuable for making drug selection for some drugs (see text)
Foot rot—cattle	No	No	No breakpoints approved for cattle or for the commonly isolated bacteria
Foot rot—sheep	+/−	No	No breakpoints approved for sheep or for the commonly isolated bacteria
Other systemic infections	Yes	+/−	May be helpful to inform drug selection (see text)

(*Enterobacterales* and macrolides). Although AST results may not be useful or necessary for some drugs for a particular bacterial species, laboratories may choose to report all antimicrobials tested; when commercial panels are used for testing (with fixed antimicrobials), drugs may be reported that are not likely to be useful. However, if a bacterial species is generally susceptible to a drug such as penicillin, the laboratory may choose *not* to perform any AST, if the drug is commonly used and available.

There are reports of some limitations of AST even when cattle-specific breakpoints are available for the bacterial species. In one report, AST of respiratory disease isolates did not provide complete prediction of clinical outcomes of metaphylaxis of tulathromycin in high-risk heifers.[11] However, in that study, the isolates were recovered from deep nasopharyngeal swabs, all susceptible isolates were from premetaphylaxis samples, and all resistant isolates were isolated from postmetaphylaxis but all the isolates were pooled in the final analysis. There are also reports of discordance between resistance based on breakpoints vs. the presence of resistance genes in mastitis organisms, suggesting a lack of predictive ability of breakpoints for clinical outcome.[12] Additional research is needed to verify these results, as the process for developing and approving breakpoints has changed considerably since the first veterinary breakpoints were approved in 1999.

HOW TO INTERPRET ANTIMICROBIAL SUSCEPTIBILITY TESTING REPORTS

Several factors affect the drugs included on diagnostic laboratory reports. Drugs included typically have one or more of the following features:

- approved cattle-specific breakpoints for categorizing isolates as susceptible or resistant,
- approved by regulatory authorities for use in cattle,
- commonly used extralabel in cattle, and
- are surrogates for a class of antimicrobial drugs to indicate susceptibility or resistance to all drugs in the class.

However, drugs may be excluded from diagnostic reports because the bacterial isolate is intrinsically resistant or because of regulatory restrictions on the use of an antimicrobial drug/drug class.

Although there are variations among laboratories in the antimicrobials drugs typically tested for bovine bacterial isolates, commercially available plates for systemic infections include the drugs listed in **Table 4** as well as clindamycin, gentamicin, neomycin, sulfadimethoxine, trimethoprim-sulfamethoxazole, tiamulin, and tylosin.[13,14] The antimicrobial drugs included in a commonly used commercial mastitis panel include those listed for mastitis[14] in **Table 5** as well as the following:

- erythromycin—no cattle-specific breakpoints; based on systemic concentrations achievable in humans; unknown correlation with outcomes in cattle with mastitis,
- oxacillin—for detection of methicillin resistance in *Staphylococcus* isolates,
- tetracycline—approved cattle-specific breakpoints based on systemic dosing and PK/PD for systemic infections, not mastitis,
- cephalothin—might be used as a surrogate for first-generation cephalosporin susceptibility, although this has not been demonstrated in clinical studies in cattle, and
- sulfadimethoxine—no cattle-specific breakpoints; based on systemic concentrations achievable in humans; unknown correlation with outcomes in cattle with mastitis.

CLSI makes freely available the current approved breakpoints for isolates from animals[15] and humans.[16] **Table 5** lists drugs that are approved for use in the United States or are legal to use extralabel for which breakpoints are approved for bacteria isolated from cattle as of 2020, including drugs used systematically and intramammary. An update is expected in late 2022, so the website should be reviewed for changes or addition. A few drugs approved in other countries but not in the United States have established breakpoints but are not provided in this table.

Of critical importance to veterinarians reviewing AST data is the dosage regimen for each breakpoint. In the VET01S document, dosage regimens are listed in Appendix D, which can be viewed freely online and should be consulted regularly to ensure the same regimen is being used in clinical practice.[15] In addition, the lack of approved breakpoints is *not* an indication of a lack of clinical effectiveness of other antimicrobials. This absence only indicates that CLSI has not been presented with data to approve breakpoints for other drugs, the bacterial organisms do not grow well in culture, there are no standardized methods for growing those bacteria, or there are not well-defined PK/PD targets for the drug.

Drugs that are commonly tested by diagnostic laboratories on isolates from cattle and small ruminants are listed in **Table 5**. This table also outlines the authors' opinions on the applicability of cattle-approved breakpoints to other clinically relevant bacteria that do not have breakpoints. It should be noted that extrapolation of breakpoints to other bacterial isolates generally lacks data to support predictions regarding clinical outcome. In addition and importantly, *these rankings are not meant to imply anything about the clinical effectiveness* but only of the applicability of breakpoints and interpretation of AST for these drugs and hosts. One exception is for surrogate drug testing, such as ampicillin, which is assumed to also predict outcomes with amoxicillin (although amoxicillin is not commonly used in the United States in cattle). It is also important to recognize that there is little evidence to support the extrapolation of clinical success with one macrolide drug to another. In addition, the drug regimen (dose, route, frequency, and duration) is critical to the interpretation of AST data, and the breakpoints approved for tetracycline as a surrogate for oxytetracycline only apply

Table 4
Antimicrobial drugs for which there are cattle-specific breakpoints approved by Clinical and Laboratory Standards Institute for systemic infections and mastitis

Antimicrobial	Body Site	Bacterial Organism(s)
Ampicillin	Metritis	E coli
	Respiratory	Mannheimia haemolytica, Pasteurella multocida, Histophilus somni
Ceftiofur	Mastitis	E coli, Staphylococcus aureus, Streptococcus agalactiae, S dysgalactiae, S uberis
	Respiratory	M haemolytica, P multocida, H somni
Danofloxacin	Respiratory	M haemolytica, P multocida
Enrofloxacin	Respiratory	M haemolytica, P multocida, H somni
Florfenicol	Respiratory	M haemolytica, P multocida, H somni
Gamithromycin	Respiratory	M haemolytica, P multocida, H somni
Penicillin G	Respiratory	M haemolytica, P multocida, H somni
Penicillin-novobiocin	Mastitis	S aureus, S agalactiae, S dysgalactiae, S uberis
Pirlimycin	Mastitis	S aureus, S agalactiae, S dysgalactiae, S uberis
Spectinomycin	Respiratory	M haemolytica, P multocida, H somni
Tetracycline (as a surrogate for oxytetracycline)	Respiratory	M haemolytica, P multocida, H somni
Tildipirosin	Respiratory	M haemolytica, P multocida, H somni
Tilmicosin	Respiratory	M haemolytica
Tulathromycin	Respiratory	M haemolytica, P multocida, H somni

to the systemic administration of long-acting oxytetracycline and *not* to any feed or water formulations of chlortetracycline and oxytetracycline. It should also be noted that the penicillin breakpoints are based on extralabel dosing.[10]

BREAKPOINTS APPROVED FOR SHEEP AND GOATS

There are no CLSI-approved breakpoints for sheep or goats for any bacterial species or drugs. Many diagnostic laboratories use cattle/swine-specific AST panels for testing isolates from sheep and goats, and some laboratories may also use the cattle-specific breakpoints for interpretation. However, caution is advised when evaluating these interpretations. Suggested interpretations are included in **Table 6** and are based on a cursory assessment of published PK data. For additional details, readers are encouraged to review VET09[10] and to consult with a clinical microbiologist or clinical pharmacologist.

As for isolates from cases of small ruminant mastitis, it is unknown how to extrapolate from cattle-specific breakpoints, given the differences in PK and the challenges of ascertaining the appropriate PK/PD target to predict clinical outcomes in sheep and goats with mastitis. Differences in PK are particularly problematic if AST is interpreted with cattle-specific breakpoints for mastitis, which are mainly based on intramammary therapy, if the animals are being treated with systemic therapy. Breakpoints should, therefore, not be applied with any confidence for small ruminant mastitis. However, if the mastitis is resulting in systemic disease that is treated via systemic therapy, the systemic breakpoints are more likely to apply, and **Table 6** could be consulted.

Table 5
Commonly tested antimicrobial drugs and the applicability of breakpoints for systemic disease in body systems without barriers to diffusion[a] to bacteria isolated from cattle

Antimicrobial Drug	Species Source for Breakpoints[b]	Gram-Positive Aerobes	Pasteurellaceae	Enterobacterales	Anaerobes
Ampicillin	Cattle	B	A	A (metritis) F (enteric disease)	D
Ceftiofur	Cattle	B	A	B	D
Cephalothin	Humans or dogs	F	F	F	F
Danofloxacin	Cattle	Illegal in the United States	A	Illegal in the United States	Illegal in the United States
Enrofloxacin	Cattle	Illegal in the United States	A	Illegal in the United States	Illegal in the United States
Erythromycin	Humans	F	F	F	F
Florfenicol	Cattle	B	A	B	B
Gamithromycin	Cattle	F	A	F	F
Gentamicin	Humans	F	F	F	F
Neomycin	Humans	F	F	F	F
Oxacillin	Humans	B	N/A	N/A	N/A
Penicillin G	Cattle	B	A	F	B
Spectinomycin	Cattle	F	A	F	F
Sulfadimethoxine	Humans	F	F	F	F
Tetracycline (as a surrogate for oxytetracycline)	Cattle	B	A	B	B
Tildipirosin	Cattle	F	A	F	F
Tilmicosin	Cattle	F	A	F	F
Trimethoprim-sulfamethoxazole	Humans	F	F	F	F
Tulathromycin	Cattle	F	A	F	F
Tylosin	[c]	F	F	F	F

Drugs are listed alphabetically as sometimes reported by diagnostic laboratories. Confidence in the applicability of the breakpoint is ranked from A to F, where A, based on cattle-approved breakpoints; C, cautiously applicable, and F, no data to support a ranking so confidence is zero or unknown. This does not include drugs for which there are approved breakpoints for mastitis, which are tissue-specific and regimen-specific.

[a] Barriers to diffusion include protected sites such as the brain as well as sequestered bone fragments, abscesses, biofilms, or foreign bodies.
[b] May need to check with diagnostic laboratory for which breakpoints are being applied by the laboratory.
[c] Breakpoints have not been established, only quality control ranges for the laboratory.

Table 6
Ranking of applicability of cattle-approved breakpoints to bacteria isolated from sheep and goats from systemic infections

Antimicrobial Drug	Sheep	Goats
Ampicillin	B	C
Ceftiofur	B	B
Danofloxacin	Illegal in the United States	Illegal in the United States
Enrofloxacin	Illegal in the United States	Illegal in the United States
Florfenicol	C	C
Gamithromycin	B	F
Penicillin G	B	B
Tetracycline (as a surrogate for oxytetracycline)	B	B
Tildipirosin	B	C
Tilmicosin	B	Lethal to goats
Tulathromycin	B	B

Drugs are listed alphabetically as sometimes reported by diagnostic laboratories. Confidence in the applicability of the breakpoint is ranked from A to F, where A, based on cattle-approved break-points, C, cautiously applicable, and F, no data to support a ranking so confidence is zero or unknown. These are not applicable to isolates from mastitis. For antimicrobial drugs without cattle-specific breakpoints, see **Table 5** for ranking estimates for cattle that could then be applied to AST results from isolates from sheep and goats.

WHAT IF YOU HAVE LIMITED CONFIDENCE IN BREAKPOINTS BUT YOU HAVE AN MIC: USING EPIDEMIOLOGIC CUTOFF VALUES FOR IDENTIFYING RESISTANCE

ECOFFs or ECVs, or epidemiological cutoff values, are not the same as breakpoints and should not be used interchangeably. However, ECOFFs may help identify isolates with resistance phenotypes that are unlikely to respond to antimicrobial therapy. An ECOFF is the MIC that separate the wild-type bacterial isolates, that is, those with no acquired resistance mechanisms, from the isolates that have acquired genes that confer resistance to the antimicrobial drug (see **Fig. 1** for a representative graph of ECOFF determination). ECOFFs are different from clinical breakpoints because they do not consider PK/PD integration or clinical outcome data. EUCAST, the European Committee on Antimicrobial Susceptibility Testing, maintains a freely available database of ECOFFs of many bacterial organisms.[17] This database can be searched by antimicrobial drug and bacterial organism that have been collected from multiple sources and therefore often represent large populations of isolates. This makes ECOFFs a potential source of information about the likelihood of a particular bacterial species carrying a resistance gene, which may be useful in "ruling-out" antimicrobials that may not be effective. Veterinarians are encouraged to consult with a clinical microbiologist or pharmacologist when using these types of data to make clinical predictions.

USING PUBLISHED ANTIMICROBIAL SUSCEPTIBILITY TESTING DATA FOR EMPIRICAL DECISION-MAKING

Although case-specific AST can be very useful, there are several reasons to select an antimicrobial empirically, that is, with only a presumptive diagnosis of bacterial disease (or a diagnosis based on criteria other than culture such as cytology), or while waiting for AST to be performed. In those instances, although the generally described spectrum of antimicrobial drugs may be helpful, such as those described in pharmacology textbooks or drug monographs, having historical data from multiple prior cases can be used to guide empirical therapy. Historical data can come from several sources:

- Antibiograms
  - From diagnostic laboratories,
  - From a production unit, clinic, or hospital, and
  - Veterinary clinics or groups of clinics might consider developing a process to create their own antibiograms; available resources provide methods to do this, which is beyond the scope of this article.[18–20]
- Drug labels
  - Package inserts and Freedom of Information summaries sometimes contain reports of bacterial isolates that were obtained during clinical trials.
- Peer-reviewed published reports
  - Searches of PubMed and other peer-reviewed literature database often reveal multiple sources of published data on populations of isolates, such as reports from diagnostic laboratories, teaching hospitals, or animal health company surveillance programs.[21–23]

When interpreting cumulative AST results, data may be presented in a variety of ways. In typical antibiograms, percent susceptible may be the only reported number for each bacterial organism/antimicrobial drug combination. In publications, the ideal presentation of data is number of isolates at each dilution of antimicrobial tested, with breakpoints indicated. With either approach, an important critical review would include an understanding of which laboratory methods were used and which breakpoints were used to categorize the isolates. If the breakpoints are not cattle-specific or approved by a standard setting body such as CLSI, caution is recommended. Other caveats would include the following:

- What region of the country or world are the animals from? How are duplicate submissions from a single premise handled?
- What body sites are included? In many cases, whether an antibiogram or publication, isolates from multiple body sites are combined, which may be misleading.
- What sampling strategy was used to collect isolates? Are they convenience samples from sick animals that may have been treated before sample collection, or from animals that died that might represent a biased subset, or from nonresponders?

These should all be considered when applying results from antibiograms, drug labels, or published articles to clinical cases.

WHAT ABOUT GENOMIC TESTING FOR ANTIMICROBIAL SUSCEPTIBILITY TESTING?

As the science of antimicrobial resistance evolves, and genetic and genomic tools improve in speed, accuracy, and price, novel approaches to predicting clinical outcomes faster are being introduced and validated.[24] Known resistance genes can be targeted with diagnostic tests and whole genome sequencing, so it seems logical to use those methods rather than traditional AST with its longer turnaround time. However, it is important to recognize that genomic methods have in general not been validated in clinical settings. They also are only able to identify known resistance genes, so if novel or unrecognized genes appear, the only way to identify them will be the phenotypic methods used in traditional AST: how much drug does it take to inhibit the growth of a bacterial isolate? Veterinarians should be extremely cautious of the promise of fast results from genomic testing, especially if the biological samples used are likely to contain organisms that are not pathogenic. Many of the genomic methods only look for genes, rather than associating those genes with a pathogenic organism. It would be inappropriate to select an antimicrobial based on the apparent resistance of a nontarget organism.

CLINICS CARE POINTS

- Breakpoints are specific to the standardized in vitro test method. Altering the test method to mimic in vivo conditions means that the breakpoints no longer apply.
- Breakpoints are specific to the antimicrobial, pathogen, host species, disease condition, and dosing regimen. Extrapolating outside of these conditions means that the correlation to clinical outcome has not been evaluated.

SUMMARY

AST is an important part of antimicrobial stewardship. Understanding how AST methods, interpretive criteria, and breakpoints are established leads to better decision-making and interpretation of AST results from bacterial isolates form cattle, sheep, and goats.

DISCLOSURE

Dr Fajt serves on various working groups of the Clinical and Laboratory Standards Institute–Veterinary Antimicrobial Susceptibility Testing subcommittee and has consulted for Tyson Foods. She has funding from the Dog Aging Project (U19 grant AG057377 from the National Institute on Aging, a part of the National Institutes of Health) and USDA Higher Education Challenge Grant 2020-70003-30927. Dr Lubbers is the current chairholder of the Clinical and Laboratory Standards Institute–Veterinary Antimicrobial Susceptibility Testing subcommittee. Dr Lubbers has also received consulting fees and/or speaker honoraria from the following: Bayer Animal Health, Boehringer Ingelheim Vetmedica, Food and Agricultural Organization of the United Nations (FAO)—Region of Asia and the Pacific, Genome Prairie, Merck Animal Health, Zoetis. No funding was received relative to the accompanying study.

REFERENCES

1. Barr FS, Carman PE, Clarkson TB. Resistance of calf scour-producing organisms to broad spectrum antibiotics. Am J Vet Res 1955;16(61 Part 1):515–6.
2. AVMA. Antimicrobial stewardship definition and core principles. American Veterinary Medical Association. Available at: https://www.avma.org/resources-tools/avma-policies/antimicrobial-stewardship-definition-and-core-principles. Accessed July 13, 2022.
3. AABP. Key elements for implementing antimicrobial stewardship plans in bovine veterinary practices working with beef and dairy operations. Available at: http://aabp.org/resources/AABP_Guidelines/AntimicrobialStewardship0322Final.pdf. Accessed July 13, 2022.
4. AASRP. Antimicrobial stewardship guidelines. Available at: http://aasrp.org/about/guidelines/AASRPantimicrobial3F.pdf. Accessed July 13, 2022.

5. CLSI. VET02Ed4 | Development of quality control ranges, breakpoints, and inter-pretive categories for antimicrobial agents used in veterinary medicine, 4th edi-tion. 2021. Available at: https://clsi.org/standards/products/veterinary-medicine/documents/vet02/. Accessed July 13, 2022.

6. Paulin A, Schneider M, Dron F, et al. Pharmacokinetic/pharmacodynamic evalua-tion of marbofloxacin as a single injection for Pasteurellaceae respiratory infec-tions in cattle using population pharmacokinetics and Monte Carlo simulations. J Vet Pharmacol Ther 2018;41(1):39–50.

7. Lees P, Potter T, Pelligand L, et al. Pharmacokinetic-pharmacodynamic integra-tion and modelling of oxytetracycline for the calf pathogens Mannheimia haemo-lytica and Pasteurella multocida. J Vet Pharmacol Ther 2018;41(1):28–38.

8. Papich MG, Lindeman C. Cephalexin susceptibility breakpoint for veterinary iso-lates: clinical Laboratory Standards Institute revision. J Vet Diagn Invest 2018; 30(1):113–20.

9. Xiao X, Chen X, Yan K, et al. PK/PD integration and pharmacodynamic cutoff of cefquinome against cow mastitis due to Escherichia coli. J Vet Pharmacol Ther 2022;45(1):83–91.

10. CLSI. VET09Ed1 | understanding susceptibility test data as a component of anti-microbial stewardship in veterinary settings, 1st Edition. Clinical & Laboratory Standards Institute. Available at: https://clsi.org/standards/products/veterinary-medicine/documents/vet09/. Accessed July 13, 2022.

11. Sarchet JJ, Pollreisz JP, Bechtol DT, et al. Limitations of bacterial culture, viral PCR, and tulathromycin susceptibility from upper respiratory tract samples in predicting clinical outcome of tulathromycin control or treatment of bovine respi-ratory disease in high-risk feeder heifers. PLoS One 2022;17(2):e0247213.

12. Ruegg PL, Oliveira L, Jin W, et al. Phenotypic antimicrobial susceptibility and occurrence of selected resistance genes in gram-positive mastitis pathogens iso-lated from Wisconsin dairy cows. J Dairy Sci 2015;98(7):4521–34.

13. ThermoFisher Scientific. Sensititre-Bovine-BOPO7F-Product-Overview-EN.pdf. Sensititre Bovine BOPO7F Product Overview. Available at: https://assets.thermofisher.com/TFS-Assets/MBD/brochures/Sensititre-Bovine-BOPO7F-Product-Overview-EN.pdf. Accessed July 13, 2022.

14. ThermoFisher Scientific. Sensititre-plate-guide-booklet-EN.pdf. Available at: https://assets.thermofisher.com/TFS-Assets/MBD/brochures/Sensititre-Plate-Guide-Booklet-EN.pdf. Accessed July 13, 2022.

15. CLSI. VET01S Free Portal. Available at: http://clsivet.org/Login.aspx. Accessed July 13, 2022.

16. CLSI. Welcome to CLSI M100 and M60. Available at: http://em100.edaptivedocs.net/Login.aspx?_ga=2.60252205.16060738.1657731650-472922369.1652734973. Accessed July 13, 2022.

17. EUCAST. MIC EUCAST. Available at: https://mic.eucast.org/. Accessed July 15, 2022.

18. Frey E, Jacob M. Development of a method for creating antibiograms for use in companion animal private practices. J Am Vet Med Assoc 2020;257(9):950–60.

19. Frey E, Jacob M. Commentary: Using antibiograms to promote antimicrobial stewardship during treatment of bacterial cystitis and superficial bacterial follic-ulitis in companion animal practice. J Am Vet Med Assoc 2020;257(9):900–3.

20. CLSI. M39Ed5 | Analysis and Presentation of Cumulative Antimicrobial Suscepti-bility Test Data, 5th Edition. Available at: https://clsi.org/standards/products/microbiology/documents/m39/. Accessed July 15, 2022.

21. Awosile BB, Heider LC, Saab ME, et al. Antimicrobial resistance in mastitis, respiratory and enteric bacteria isolated from ruminant animals from the Atlantic Provinces of Canada from 1994-2013. Can Vet J Rev Veterinaire Can 2018; 59(10):1099–104.

22. Berge ACB, Moore DA, Sischo WM. Prevalence and antimicrobial resistance patterns of Salmonella enterica in preweaned calves from dairies and calf ranches. Am J Vet Res 2006;67(9):1580–8.

23. Sweeney M, Gunnett L, Mohan Kumar D, et al. Antimicrobial susceptibility of Actinobacillus pleuropneumoniae, Bordetella bronchiseptica, Pasteurella multocida, and Streptococcus suis isolated from diseased pigs in the United States and Canada, 2016 to 2020. J Swine Health Prod 2022;30(3):130–44.

24. Hesp A, Veldman K, Brouwer MSM, et al. Latent class analysis to assess whole-genome sequencing versus broth microdilution for monitoring antimicrobial resistance in livestock. Prev Vet Med 2021;193(cwt, 8217463):105406.

Diagnostics for Viral Pathogens in Veterinary Diagnostic Laboratories

Leyi Wang, DVM, PhD, DACVM

KEYWORDS

- Viral diagnostics • Active infection • Serological responses • Virus isolation
- Antigen test • PCR • ELISA • Serum neutralization

KEY POINTS

- Diagnostics for viral pathogens include testing for both viral active infection and serological responses to viruses.
- Identifying viral active infection can be accomplished via virus isolation, electron microscopy, viral antigen tests, and molecular polymerase chain reaction. Initial identification followed by further whole genome sequencing is key to characterizing any strain involved in an outbreak scenario.
- Serological tests are used for measuring previous exposure to viruses or vaccination efficacy.

INTRODUCTION

Viruses are obligate parasites requiring the use of host machinery for replication. Different from other microbes such as bacteria, viruses therefore rely on host cells to survive. Viral hosts include plants, animals, bacteria, and archaea. In the case of animals, viruses play a crucial role in the pathogenesis of different types of infectious disease syndromes including respiratory, enteric, neurological, and urogenital infections. A few viruses in the families *Retroviridae*, *Papillomaviridae*, *Herpesviridae*, and *Adenoviridae* can also cause neoplasia and tumors in animals.

Diagnostic investigation of viral infectious diseases needs to include consideration of multiple factors including clinical presentation, gross lesions, microscopic lesions, and laboratory antigen and/or antibody testing. Laboratory testing is just one component of definitive diagnosis and a negative test result does not exclude the possibility of an infection with the specific pathogen of interest. Patient selection, sample selection, sample timing, sample quality, test selection, and laboratory processing all could

Disclosure: None.
Department of Veterinary Clinical Medicine, Veterinary Diagnostic Laboratory, College of Veterinary Medicine, University of Illinois at Urbana-Champaign, 2001 South Lincoln Avenue, VMBSB Room 1222A, Urbana, IL 61802, USA
E-mail address: leyiwang@illinois.edu

Vet Clin Food Anim 39 (2023) 129–140
https://doi.org/10.1016/j.cvfa.2022.09.002
0749-0720/23/© 2022 Elsevier Inc. All rights reserved.
vetfood.theclinics.com

Abbreviations	
VI	virus isolation
EM	electron microscopy
ELISA	antigen enzyme-linked immunoassay
ICA	immunochromatographic assay
DFA	direct fluorescent antibody test
PCR	polymerase chain reaction
IFA	indirect fluorescent antibody test
AGID	agar gel immunodiffusion assay
SN	serum neutralization
HI	hemagglutination inhibition

affect the significance of a test result. Laboratory testing for viruses in animals is generally divided into 2 categories: detection of active infection and detection of previous exposure (**Fig. 1**). Assays used for detection of an ongoing infection include virus isolation (VI), electron microscopy (EM), antigen enzyme-linked immunoassay (ELISA), immunochromatographic assay (ICA), direct fluorescent antibody test (DFA), and polymerase chain reaction (PCR). Tests used for detection of previous exposure include antibody ELISA, indirect fluorescent antibody test (IFA), agar gel immunodiffusion assay (AGID), and serum neutralization (SN) (see **Fig. 1**). Hemagglutination inhibition (HI) serological assay can be also performed for viruses with hemagglutination characteristics.

SAMPLE COLLECTION

Samples can include multiple types such as swab samples from syndrome relevant anatomical locations or areas of pathophysiological reaction (nasal, oral,

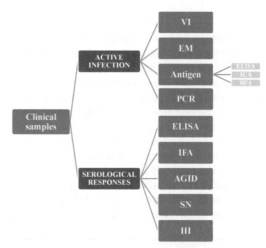

Fig. 1. The diagram shows tests commonly used for detecting active viral infection and serological responses to viruses. Tests for active infection include VI, EM, antigen tests, and PCR; assays for detection of serological responses to viruses include ELISA, IFA, AGID, SN, and HI. Antigen tests have antigen ELISA, ICA, and DFA. AGID, and agar gel immunodiffusion assay. DFA, direct fluorescent antibody test; ELISA, antigen enzyme-linked immunoassay; EM, electron microscopy; HI, Hemagglutination inhibition; ICA, immunochromatographic assay; IFA, indirect fluorescent antibody test; PCR, polymerase chain reaction; SN, serum neutralization; VI, virus isolation.

nasopharyngeal, oropharyngeal, tracheal, conjunctival, lachrymal, ocular, vesical, fecal, cloacal), tracheal wash, broncho-alveolar lavage, EDTA-blood, urine, cerebrospinal fluid, oral fluid, vesicular fluid, effusion fluid (ascites, pleural), serum, semen, milk, ear notch, skin scrapings, and other different tissues (**Table 1**). Flocked, foam, spun polyester (eg, dacron), and spun rayon tipped swabs can be used in sample collection for viral testing. Flocked swab is preferred superior than nonflocked as previously reported.[1] Calcium alginate swabs and swabs with wooden handle should be avoided for sample collection because of potential interference with viral testing. Swabs are collected into viral transport media such as brain heart infusion broth or saline like phosphate buffered saline. Among those sample types, oral fluid is commonly used in pig testing because cotton ropes hung in pig farms are easy to manipulate and oral fluids can be used for the evaluation of pig herds at the population or subpopulation level. Fresh ear notch samples can be collected using a commercial ear notcher and are commonly used for testing bovine viral diarrhea virus (BVDV) persistent infection by an antigen ELISA or pooled for PCR testing in cattle. Freshly collected samples can be shipped to the diagnostic laboratories with ice packs for overnight delivery.

DETECTION OF VIRAL ACTIVE INFECTION

Methods used for detecting viral active infection have lower (VI, EM) and higher (antigen test and PCR) specificity to particular viruses of interest, and their sensitivity of detecting viruses range from low to high in the order of EM, VI, antigen test, and PCR (**Fig. 2**).[2,3] A negative result does not exclude the possibility of animal infected with a virus of interest. Reasons for false-negative testing results include low sample

Type	Name
Table 1 **Different types of samples used for clinical viral testing**	
Swabs	Nasal
	Nasopharyngeal
	Oral
	Oropharyngeal
	Tracheal
	Conjunctival
	Lachrymal
	Ocular
	Vesical
	Fecal
	Cloacal
Fluids	Tracheal wash
	Broncho-alveolar lavage
	EDTA-blood
	Urine
	Cerebrospinal fluid
	Oral fluid
	Vesicular fluid
	Effusion fluid (ascites, pleural)
	Serum
	Semen
	Milk
Other	Ear notch
	Skin scrapings
	All types of tissues

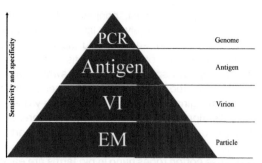

Fig. 2. Standardized hierarchical tests for detecting active viral infection. From bottom to top with increasing sensitivity and specificity. Their targets of EM, VI, antigen, and PCR are viral particle, infectious virion, viral antigen, and viral genome, respectively. EM, electron microscopy; PCR, polymerase chain reaction; VI, virus isolation.

quality, nonoptimal sample type, improper sample timing (missed the window period for testing active infection, too early or too late), low sensitivity of the assay used, and/ or to a too high of specificity test used (new variants missed due to mutations in target sequences).

Virus Isolation

VI was commonly used for viral testing in 1980s and 1990s and is still performed now but primarily for autogenous vaccine production and research purposes. When new viruses emerge in the field, VI is a crucial step for downstream in vivo characterization of their roles in diseases. Cell culture, embryonated chicken eggs, and even animals can be used for VI but cell culture is the most frequently used method. VI is a cell line–dependent assay. Some viruses only grow in a single type of cell line, whereas others can replicate in multiple cell lines (**Table 2**). VI is labor-intensive and time-consuming and sometimes needs several passages before cytopathic effect (CPE) are clearly visible. In addition to observation of CPE, supplemental tests such as DFA, EM, and PCR are needed to confirm specific successful VI. An example is CPE observation in MA-104 cells during VI for bovine rotavirus although rotavirus failed to be detected via PCR.[4] Further EM observation revealed the presence of viral-like particles, which were confirmed as bovine parechovirus by next-generation sequencing. In terms of BVDV, VI is normally performed using cell culture supplemented with horse serum instead of fetal bovine serum (FBS), due to potential contamination of FBS with BVDV.[5] Because of presence of 2 biotypes cytopathic (CP) and noncytopathic (NCP), VI for BVDV should be always confirmed by DFA or PCR to catch those NCP strains.

Most viruses can be isolated via cell culture but viruses in certain families such as noroviruses in the family *Caliciviridae* are difficult to isolate. For porcine reproductive and respiratory syndrome virus (PRRSV), the MARC-145 cell line is commonly used for VI but the successful isolation rate is much lower than that of ZMAC cells, which are derived from lung lavage fluid samples from porcine fetuses.[6] ZMAC cells express typical macrophage markers.[7] Probable interaction between viruses and host cells contributes to the difference between the 2 cell lines for PRRSV isolation. To improve VI efficiency, vero cells expressing dog SLAM (CD150) receptor for canine distemper virus were developed.[8] Similar increase in VI efficiency is accomplished by addition of trypsin to cell culture for some viruses such as coronaviruses.[9,10] Bile acids are required for isolation of viruses such as porcine sapovirus.[11] If coinfection by different viruses or different genotypes of a virus are present in the case, VI may propagate both viral isolates or just the predominant isolate in the sample and plaque purification is

Table 2
Cell lines used for virus isolation

Species	Virus	Cell Lines
Ruminant	Bovine respiratory syncytial virus	MDBK, BT
	Bovine viral diarrheal virus	MDBK, BT
	Parainfluenza virus 3	MDBK, BT
	Bovine herpesvirus virus 1, IBRV	MDBK, BT
	Bovine herpes virus 4	BT
	Bluetongue virus	C6/36, BHK, Vero
	Epizootic hemorrhagic disease virus	C6/36, BHK, Vero
Porcine	PRRSV	MARC-145, ZMAC, PAM
	Swine influenza virus	MDCK
	Porcine circovirus 2	PK-15
	Transmissible gastroenteritis virus	ST
	Porcine epidemic diarrhea virus	Vero
	Porcine deltacoronavirus	PK-15, ST
	Porcine parvovirus	PK-15, ST
	Porcine adenovirus	PK-15
	Senecavirus A virus	LC NCI-H1299, BHK-21
	Porcine hemagglutinating encephalomyelitis virus	HRT-18
	Encephalomyocarditis virus	BHK-21
	Porcine pseudorabies virus	PK-15
Equine	Equine herpesvirus-1	MDBK, RK13
	Equine influenza virus	MDCK
	Equine arteritis virus	RK13
Canine	Canine adenovirus	MDCK
	Canine distemper virus	Vero dog SLAM
	Canine herpesvirus	MDCK, CRFK
	Canine parvovirus	CRFK
	Canine coronavirus	MDCK, CRFK, A72
	Canine parainfluenza virus	MDCK, CRFK, A72
Feline	Feline coronavirus	CRFK
	Feline herpesvirus	CRFK
	Feline calicivirus	CRFK

Abbreviations: BHK-21, Baby Hamster Kidney 21; BT, Bovine Turbinate; CRFK, Crandell-Rees Feline Kidney Cell; HRT-18, Human Rectal Tumor-18; IBRV, Infectious Bovine Rhinotracheitis virus; LC, human lung carcinoma; MDBK, Madin-Darby bovine kidney; MDCK, Madin-Darby canine kidney; PAM, Porcine Alveolar Macrophages; PK-15, Porcine Kidney 15; RK13, Rabbit Kidney epithelial cells; ST, Swine Testicle.

needed to isolate them.[12] For coinfection by 2 types of PRRSV, ZMAC was capable of isolating both types, whereas the MARC-145 cell line only isolated one type.[13] In summary, VI has significant utility for certain diagnostic purposes such as new virus discovery; however, the caveats described above make the potential for false-negative results when used for routine testing purposes.

Electron Microscopy

Based on the size, shape, appearance of the capsid, presence or absence of an envelope, and surface projections, EM can usually identify the virus to a family or genus level using a negative staining method. Clinically, EM is more sensitive for the detection of rotavirus, coronavirus, poxvirus, and parapoxvirus compared with other virus types.[14] EM normally requires a high amount of viral particles ($\geq 10^5$ particle/mL) in the specimen,[15] which highlights its low sensitivity, and is subjective in terms of the result interpretation. Due to these drawbacks as well as the longer turnaround time and higher cost, EM is less commonly used for routine diagnostics. EM might be useful in new virus discovery, especially for those samples tested negative by routine methods. The identification of bovine parechovirus in cattle with diarrhea[4] and porcine deltacoronavirus in pigs are good examples of viruses that were discovered using EM.[16]

DETECTION OF VIRAL ANTIGEN

Three different antigen testing methods used in veterinary diagnostic laboratories are antigen ELISA, ICA, and DFA. Antigen ELISAs are available for avian influenza virus, feline leukemia virus, and BVDV in some laboratories. Antigen ELISA methods are typically lower in sensitivity than PCR or molecular-based approaches (see **Fig. 2**). Antigen ELISA for BVDV is useful in identifying persistently infected cattle with the use of skin samples ear notches but testing blood or serum samples by BVDV antigen ELISA might be complicated by the presence of maternal antibodies in young calves.[17] Therefore, calves younger than 3 months old should not be tested with BVDV antigen ELISA using serum samples.[18] ICA is another point-of-care format of test for detecting viral antigen with a quick turnaround time. A commercial ICA kit (SAS Rota test, SA Scientific, San Antonio, TX) is available for the detection of any group of rotavirus. There is also a commercial ICA kit Bovine Enterichek (Biovet) for the detection of bovine coronavirus, bovine rotavirus A, and other 2 nonviral pathogens.[19] The results of antigen ELISA are based on the optical density (OD) value, whereas those of ICA are based on visualization of specific bands. DFA is commonly used for the detection of viral antigens in tissue and blood samples in laboratories and is mainly utilized in necropsy cases. Due to the subjective nature of the results and lower sensitivity, DFA is gradually being replaced by molecular testing methods for most viruses. DFA remains a gold standard test for the detection of rabies virus in brain tissues.

Polymerase Chain Reaction

PCR is used to detect viral genomes of DNA and RNA viruses. Unlike DNA viruses, RNA viruses require and additional reverse transcription (RT) step before PCR amplification. Either conventional PCR or real-time PCR can be used for testing viral samples. Conventional PCR requires visualization of results (such as gel electrophoresis), whereas real-time PCR produces a cycle threshold (Ct), which is inversely correlated with the amount of viral genomes in a sample. A high value of Ct indicates a low viral load, which may indicate an inadequate incubation period or a convalescent stage, a nonoptimal sample type, or mismatch between sequences of primers and probes and a new variant. In general, positive PCR results do not differentiate infected from vaccinated animals since high Ct values are not always produced from animals with modified-live viral vaccines and the amount of viral genome detected can vary depending on the administered routes of vaccines.[20] If live-modified vaccine strains contain markers in the genome, PCR differentiation of vaccinated from wild type infected animals could be possible.

Because of higher sensitivity, sample pooling is used in real-time PCR testing of clinically abnormal animals that are suspected to be infected with certain viruses, such as for BVDV with ear notches or serum, PRRSV with serum, and avian influenza virus with swabs. Conventional PCR or real-time PCR is commonly used to detect not only single genomic targets of a virus but usually 2 or more targets of a single or multiple viruses for differential testing. There are duplex real-time PCRs for detecting PRRSV North American and European genotypes, porcine circovirus 2 and 3, equine herpesvirus 1 and 4, and BVDV1 and BVDV2. Syndrome-specific multiplex PCR panels exist to test for bovine respiratory viral pathogens (bovine herpesvirus 1, BVDV, bovine parainfluenza virus 3, and bovine respiratory syncytial virus)[21,22] or bovine enteric pathogens (bovine coronavirus, bovine rotavirus group A, and other 3 nonviral pathogens) in a single sample.[23]

Because real-time PCR and PCR only target partial genome of viruses, both cannot provide information about whether there are changes in the remaining regions, and additional testing such as subtyping PCR or sequencing is needed for further virus characterization. Because of its higher sensitivity, not all positive samples (especially very weak positive) by real-time PCR are suitable for further characterization by other lower sensitivity methods such as sequencing and VI. Cutoff values ($\leq$31) of positive samples for whole genome or single gene sequencing vary depending on the types of viruses, types of samples, and sequencing methods used.[24–27] For those samples with high Ct values unsuitable for sequencing, characterization by other methods including immunohistochemistry can be performed. The first example is the identification of a recombinant PRRSV strain in the United States with about 7000 nucleotides in the 5' end and remaining genome highly related to wild-type and Fostera vaccine strains, respectively.[28] Routine PRRSV real-time RT-PCR of 2 samples of a pig farm revealed the presence of a North American genotype. ORF5 sequencing identified a vaccine strain and a wild-type strain in 2 samples but vaccine-specific real-time RT-PCR for nonstructural protein 2 region was negative in both samples. In addition to the wild-type strain, whole genome sequencing confirmed the presence of a new recombinant strain between a vaccine strain and a wild-type strain. The second example is the identification of the variant porcine epidemic diarrhea virus (PEDV) in the United States. This variant strain had major changes in the spike gene that were not detected because the nucleocapsid gene was targeted in the real-time RT-PCR.[29] Clinically attenuated signs in piglets prompted further characterization of the strain using whole genome sequencing, and mutations (3 deletions, 1 insertion, and several point mutations) in the spike were observed only in the identified variant PEDV strain OH851. The last example is the identification of sparrow deltacoronavirus in the United States. Because of the high genome similarity in nonspike regions such as ORF1ab and the nucelocapsid gene between sparrow and porcine deltacoronaviruses, real-time RT-PCR designed to detect porcine deltacoronavirus also can detect sparrow deltacoronavirus. In hoop-style pig buildings with uncontrolled access for wild birds, feces of sparrows positive for sparrow deltacoronavirus might contaminate porcine samples, resulting in false-positive results for porcine deltacoronavirus in samples collected from clinically healthy pigs.[30] Therefore, whole genome sequencing is a must to characterize each specific strain and identify any changes (deletion, insertion, point mutation, recombination).

Similar to deltacoronavirus in different porcine and bird species mentioned above, bovine-like coronaviruses are present in various animal species including domestic and wild ruminants and even nonruminant animals, which could potentially complicate testing of bovine coronavirus in farm animals commingled with other animals.[31,32] Additionally, no genetic markers were found in coronaviruses causing either bovine respiratory or enteric diseases. Identification of new emerging viruses usually involves in either pan-PCR plus sequencing (such as discover of bovine Hobi-like pestivirus in China)[33] or directly metagenomic sequencing (such as the example of identification bovine parechovirus).[4] These are important considerations given the emergence of new viruses and virus strains in livestock and may be useful to investigate suspected viral disease outbreaks that have no identifiable cause.

DETECTION OF SEROLOGICAL RESPONSES TO VIRUSES

Paired serum samples collected in the acute and convalescent stages of illness can be used to determine an active infection in animals. Testing a single serum sample normally can predict previous exposure to any viruses or immune status to viruses after vaccination. Commonly used assays for serological responses are ELISA, IFA, AGID, SN, and HI. In general, positive serological results do not differentiate maternal antibodies or exposure, nor vaccine or wild type virus exposure.

ANTIBODY ENZYME-LINKED IMMUNOASSAY

Due to a quicker turnaround time and higher sensitivity, ELISA is commonly used for testing for the presence of antibodies to many viruses. Either an indirect antibody ELISA or competitive ELISA (cELISA) can be used. ELISA is primarily used as a screening test, and in some cases, the results are confirmed by alternative testing methodologies with higher specificity. For example, serum samples with positive PRRSV antibody ELISA results are further tested by IFA. Moreover, positive ELISA results of equine infectious anemia virus (EIAV) are confirmed by AGID. For reportable diseases with vaccination programs available, serological tests should be compatible with differentiation of infected from vaccinated animals. A great example is the porcine pseudorabies virus (PRV) with the development of a gene-deleted (gI/gE) "marker" vaccine. ELISA gI antibody test can be used to determine exposure to PRV field strains or vaccines containing gI antigen, whereas ELISA gB antibody test can be used to evaluate immune status or exposure to the PRV together with gI ELISA antibody test. The results of indirect antibody ELISA are evaluated directly using the OD value, or calculated as sample-to-positive ratios based on OD values, whereas the results of cELISA is calculated as the percentage inhibition using OD values of samples and negative control.

Indirect Fluorescent Antibody Test

Compared with ELISA with capability of scale-up testing, IFA is laborious and less sensitive and thus less commonly used. There are IFA assays for feline infectious peritonitis, porcine circovirus type 2, PEDV, transmissible gastroenteritis virus, and PRRSV. The results rely on the observation of fluorescent signals using a fluorescent microscope and therefore the interpretation of results is subjective. Through a serial dilution of samples, IFA can be used to semiquantitatively measure IFA titers of the samples.

Agar Gel Immunodiffusion

AGID is one of the most commonly used serological assays for viruses such as avian influenza virus, epizootic hemorrhagic disease virus, and hemorrhagic enteritis virus. The result of AGID is based on observation of the precipitin line formed between antigen and specific antibodies around 24 to 48 hours after setting up the test. Because AGID has a higher specificity than ELISA, AGID is usually used as a confirmatory test for ELISA surveillance testing of some viruses, such as EIAV.

Serum neutralization

SN, sometimes termed virus neutralization, is a serological test to measure the titer of neutralizing antibodies present in serum samples postinfection or after vaccination. Conventional SN is based on the inhibition of virus infectivity by neutralizing antibodies in cell culture and the result is to observe the absence of CPE. The SN titer is calculated as the reciprocal of the highest dilution of a serum sample that produces absence of CPE. For evaluation of immunization status, SN titers are generally correlated with protection in vivo. In some cases, SN is required for shipping animals, such as vesicular stomatitis virus. SN is technically demanding, labor-intensive, and time-consuming. Interpretation of the results relies on availability of information about vaccination history, time points of sampling, and disease history. Cattle with killed vaccine have relatively lower SN titers than those with modified-live vaccine, whereas nonvaccinated animals with wild type virus infection have relative similar or higher titers than live vaccinated animals. Additionally, SN for viruses requiring biosafety level (BSL) 3 will be unavailable for those laboratories with only access to BSL 2 facilities. In addition to conventional SN, pseudovirus neutralization assay[34] or surrogate virus neutralization test based on blockage of viral receptor and protein interaction[35] are also available.

Hemagglutination-inhibition
HI test is commonly used for those viruses in the families of *Orthomyxoviridae*, *Paramyxoviridae*, *Parvoviridae*, and *Adenoviridae* with hemagglutination characteristics capable of agglutinating erythrocytes. HI assays measure antibodies that block the viral hemagglutinin action to agglutinate erythrocytes, thus allowing erythrocytes to sink to the bottom of the well of a microtiter plate. Therefore, the HI result is based on observation of the formation of a "button" of erythrocytes at the bottom of the plate well. The HI titer is calculated as the reciprocal of the highest dilution of a serum sample that produces complete inhibition of hemagglutination.

SUMMARY

Laboratory testing is one part of clinical diagnosis and quick and reliable testing results provide important data to support treatment decision and develop control strategies. Detection of active infection and serological responses to viruses are 2 viral diagnostic approaches that complement each other because the window period for testing active infection is much shorter than that of detecting serological responses. In the past few decades, clinical viral testing has been shifting from traditional VI and EM to molecular PCR and point-of-care antigen tests. This shift in diagnostic methodology also means change from looking for infectious virions or viral particles to hunting viral antigens and genomes. Viral serological testing continues to evolve from methods that detect antibodies with a lower level of sensitivity to methods with both higher sensitivity and specificity. These changes also allow for high-throughput testing in veterinary diagnostic laboratories. With technological development, it is predicted that metagenomic sequencing will be commonly used in veterinary clinical diagnosis for unveiling the whole picture of microbes involved in diseases in the future.

CLINICS CARE POINTS

- Clinical viral testing is affected by multiple factors including sample timing, sample type, sample quality, and test methods.
- Testing for active infection has a shorter time window than for previous exposure.
- Low viral loads may indicate animals could be in either early infection or recovery stage, recently vaccinated with modified live vaccines, or samples from nonoptimal replication sites of virus.

- A negative testing result sometimes does not exclude the possibility of animals infected with viruses of interest.

REFERENCES

1. Spackman E, Pedersen JC, McKinley ET, et al. Optimal specimen collection and transport methods for the detection of avian influenza virus and Newcastle disease virus. BMC Vet Res 2013;9:35.
2. A Williams R, Savage CE, Jones RC. A comparison of direct electron microscopy, virus isolation and a DNA amplification method for the detection of avian infectious laryngotracheitis virus in field material. Avian Pathol 1994; 23:709–20.
3. Currie DW, Shah MM, Salvatore PP, et al. Relationship of SARS-CoV-2 antigen and reverse transcription PCR Positivity for Viral cultures. Emerg Infect Dis 2022;28:717–20.
4. Oba M, Sakaguchi S, Wu H, et al. First isolation and genomic characterization of bovine parechovirus from faecal samples of cattle in Japan. J Gen Virol 2022; 103(2). https://doi.org/10.1099/jgv.0.001718.
5. Evermann JF, Berry ES, Baszler TV, et al. Diagnostic approaches for the detection of bovine viral diarrhea (BVD) virus and related pestiviruses. J Vet Diagn Invest 1993;5:265–9.
6. Yim-Im W, Huang H, Park J, et al. Comparison of ZMAC and marc-145 cell lines for improving porcine reproductive and respiratory syndrome virus isolation from clinical samples. J Clin Microbiol 2021;59(3):e01757–20.
7. Calzada-Nova G, Husmann RJ, Schnitzlein WM, et al. Effect of the host cell line on the vaccine efficacy of an attenuated porcine reproductive and respiratory syndrome virus. Vet Immunol Immunopathol 2012;148:116–25.
8. Seki F, Ono N, Yamaguchi R, et al. Efficient isolation of wild strains of canine distemper virus in Vero cells expressing canine SLAM (CD150) and their adaptability to marmoset B95a cells. J Virol 2003;77:9943–50.
9. Hu H. Isolation and propagation of porcine deltacoronavirus in cell culture and embryonated chicken eggs. In: Wang L, editor. Animal coronaviruses. New York, NY: Humana; 2022. p. 103–14.
10. Wang Q. Isolation of porcine epidemic diarrhea virus from clinical samples. In: Wang L, editor. Animal coronaviruses. New York, NY: Humana; 2022. p. 87–93.
11. Chang KO, Sosnovtsev SV, Belliot G, et al. Bile acids are essential for porcine enteric calicivirus replication in association with down-regulation of signal transducer and activator of transcription 1. Proc Natl Acad Sci U S A 2004;101: 8733–8.
12. Toda S, Okamoto R, Nishida T, et al. Isolation of influenza A/H3 and B viruses from an influenza patient: confirmation of co-infection by two influenza viruses. Jpn J Infect Dis 2006;59:142–3.
13. Yim-Im W, Huang H, Zheng Y, et al. Characterization of PRRSV in clinical samples and the corresponding cell culture isolates. Transbound Emerg Dis 2022;69(5): e3045–59.
14. Naeem K, Goyal SM. Comparison of virus isolation, immunofluorescence and electron microscopy for the diagnosis of animal viruses. Microbiologica 1988; 11:355–62.
15. Nitsche A, Gelderblom HR, Eisendle K, et al. Pitfalls in diagnosing human poxvirus infections. J Clin Virol 2007;38:165–8.

16. Wang L, Byrum B, Zhang Y. Detection and genetic characterization of deltacoronavirus in pigs, Ohio, USA, 2014. Emerg Infect Dis 2014;20:1227–30.
17. Hilbe M, Stalder H, Peterhans E, et al. Comparison of five diagnostic methods for detecting bovine viral diarrhea virus infection in calves. J Vet Diagn Invest 2007; 19:28–34.
18. Zimmer GM, Van Maanen C, De Goey I, et al. The effect of maternal antibodies on the detection of bovine virus diarrhoea virus in peripheral blood samples. Vet Microbiol 2004;100:145–9.
19. Cho YI, Sun D, Cooper V, et al. Evaluation of a commercial rapid test kit for detecting bovine enteric pathogens in feces. J Vet Diagn Invest 2012;24:559–62.
20. Walz PH, Newcomer BW, Riddell KP, et al. Virus detection by PCR following vaccination of naive calves with intranasal or injectable multivalent modified-live viral vaccines. J Vet Diagn Invest 2017;29:628–35.
21. Thonur L, Maley M, Gilray J, et al. One-step multiplex real time RT-PCR for the detection of bovine respiratory syncytial virus, bovine herpesvirus 1 and bovine parainfluenza virus 3. BMC Vet Res 2012;8:37.
22. Horwood PF, Mahony TJ. Multiplex real-time RT-PCR detection of three viruses associated with the bovine respiratory disease complex. J Virol Methods 2011; 171:360–3.
23. Cho YI, Kim WI, Liu S, et al. Development of a panel of multiplex real-time polymerase chain reaction assays for simultaneous detection of major agents causing calf diarrhea in feces. J Vet Diagn Invest 2010;22:509–17.
24. Zhang J, Zheng Y, Xia XQ, et al. High-throughput whole genome sequencing of Porcine reproductive and respiratory syndrome virus from cell culture materials and clinical specimens using next-generation sequencing technology. J Vet Diagn Invest 2017;29:41–50.
25. Paden CR, Tao Y, Queen K, et al. Rapid, Sensitive, Full-Genome Sequencing of Severe Acute Respiratory Syndrome Coronavirus 2. Emerg Infect Dis 2020;26: 2401–5.
26. Guzman M, Melendez R, Jimenez C, et al. Analysis of ORF5 sequences of porcine reproductive and respiratory syndrome virus (PRRSV) circulating within swine farms in Costa Rica. BMC Vet Res 2021;17:217.
27. Lewandowski K, Xu Y, Pullan ST, et al. Metagenomic nanopore sequencing of influenza virus direct from clinical respiratory samples. J Clin Microbiol 2019;58.
28. Wang A, Chen Q, Wang L, et al. Recombination between vaccine and field strains of porcine reproductive and respiratory syndrome virus. Emerg Infect Dis 2019; 25:2335–7.
29. Wang L, Byrum B, Zhang Y. New variant of porcine epidemic diarrhea virus, United States, 2014. Emerg Infect Dis 2014;20:917–9.
30. Chen Q, Wang L, Yang C, et al. The emergence of novel sparrow deltacoronaviruses in the United States more closely related to porcine deltacoronaviruses than sparrow deltacoronavirus HKU17. Emerg Microbes Infect 2018;7:105.
31. Savard C, Provost C, Ariel O, et al. First report and genomic characterization of a bovine-like coronavirus causing enteric infection in an odd-toed non-ruminant species (Indonesian tapir, Acrocodia indica) during an outbreak of winter dysentery in a zoo. Transbound Emerg Dis 2021;69(5):3056–65.
32. Amer HM. Bovine-like coronaviruses in domestic and wild ruminants. Anim Health Res Rev 2018;19:113–24.
33. Chen M, Liu M, Liu S, et al. HoBi-like pestivirus infection leads to bovine death and severe respiratory disease in China. Transbound Emerg Dis 2021;68: 1069–74.

34. Tolah AMK, Sohrab SS, Tolah KMK, et al. Evaluation of a pseudovirus neutralization assay for SARS-CoV-2 and correlation with live virus-based micro neutralization assay. Diagnostics (Basel) 2021;11(6):994.
35. Tan CW, Chia WN, Qin X, et al. A SARS-CoV-2 surrogate virus neutralization test based on antibody-mediated blockage of ACE2-spike protein-protein interaction. Nat Biotechnol 2020;38:1073–8.

Serology in Bovine Infectious Disease Diagnosis

Amelia R. Woolums, DVM, MVSc, PhD

KEYWORDS

- ELISA • Serum neutralization • Seroconversion • Titer • Paired serology • Cattle
- Calves

KEY POINTS

- Serology can help to confirm past infection or vaccination but misunderstanding the significance of serologic results can lead to diagnostic errors.
- To aid the interpretation of serologic results, think about whether antibodies were induced by an agent causing permanent infection, transient infection with no history of vaccination, or transient infection with possible vaccination.
- When serology is used to identify evidence of infection in cattle that have been vaccinated, paired serologic testing of multiple animals, using samples collected 2 to 4 weeks apart, provides the best chance for informative results.
- Serologic testing to diagnose infection in calves expected to have maternal antibodies can be difficult to interpret; serologic testing may be most clearly informative if used only in cattle not expected to have maternal antibodies.

SEROLOGY: HOW DOES IT WORK?
Definition

Serology is the measurement of antibodies to specific infectious agents in serum from one or more individuals, to determine whether they have been infected with, or vaccinated against, those agents. Serology is often used to diagnose an infectious cause of disease, to guide therapy and future preventive efforts, but it can also be used to assess the effect of vaccination schemes, or for disease surveillance in populations. Serology can also be used to determine whether calves acquired passive immunity from colostrum to specific agents, although in most cases total immunoglobulin G (IgG) directed against all agents (or a surrogate marker, eg, serum total protein) is measured to assess transfer of passive immunity. Although the term "serology" most precisely refers to the evaluation of serum, testing other types of

Dr A.R. Woolums has received funding for research and consulting from companies that manufacture and market vaccines for administration to cattle.
Department of Pathobiology and Population Medicine, Mississippi State University, Mississippi State, MS 39762, USA
E-mail address: amelia.woolums@msstate.edu

Vet Clin Food Anim 39 (2023) 141–155
https://doi.org/10.1016/j.cvfa.2022.10.007
vetfood.theclinics.com

samples for antibodies to specific agents, such as whole blood, saliva, or nasal secretions, for the purposes indicated above, can also be considered a type of serologic diagnosis.

Basic Principles of Serology

In serology, antibodies directed against specific agents (ie, "antigen-specific" or "agent-specific" antibodies) are measured, in contrast to the measurement of total antibodies, which may be done to characterize general host humoral immune capability, or to assess transfer of passive immunity. Antibodies are also known as "immunoglobulins," and cattle produce five immunoglobulin classes (or "isotypes"): IgG, IgM, IgA, IgE, and IgD.[1] Therefore, agent-specific antibodies can include molecules in all five classes. Note that IgD is expressed almost entirely on the surface of B cells, and IgE is mostly attached to the surface of mast cells and eosinophils in tissues via the Fc epsilon receptor on those cells–although small amounts of antigen-specific IgD and IgE can be measured in bovine serum.[1] Thus, when serologic testing is used to measure antibodies to a specific agent in serum or other body fluid, the antibodies being measured will almost entirely be IgG, IgM, and/or IgA. However, when samples are sent to a veterinary diagnostic laboratory for serologic testing to identify antibodies to specific infectious agents, the laboratory usually does not identify the antibody class. Although tests to specifically measure IgG, IgM, or IgA could be requested, most veterinary diagnostic laboratories do not offer tests to measure specific antibody classes against specific infectious agents; such tests are usually reserved for research applications.

In bovine serum, the antibody class present in the highest concentration is IgG (IgG1 > IgG2), then IgM, then IgA. IgM is the first antibody produced in response to infection or vaccination, and after a primary infection or vaccination, IgM can be identified in serum within 5 to 9 days after exposure and is present for approximately 4 to 8 weeks (**Fig. 1**). IgG is produced next, and after a primary infection or vaccination, is first identified in serum approximately 14 to 21 days later and is present for several weeks. In response to second and subsequent future exposures, IgM will again be produced first, but IgG will be detectable sooner, and the concentration of IgG will be much higher, than after the primary response (see **Fig. 1**). These times are

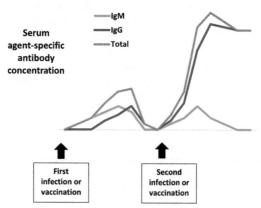

Fig. 1. Relative changes in serum infectious agent-specific IgM, IgG, and total antibody over time after an individual receives the first (primary) and second infection with, or vaccination against, an infectious agent. Agent-specific serum IgA or IgE, which may be measurable are not shown.

approximations; the exact timing of specific antibody appearance and duration in an individual will vary depending on factors related to the nature of the infection or vaccine exposure, and factors related to the host immune response. Examples of the changes in serum agent-specific antibody classes over time in calves exposed to two bovine pathogens are demonstrated in **Tables 1** and **2**.[2,3] The relevance of this information is that if antibody is measured by an assay that does not distinguish specific classes, serum antibody measured within the first week or two after a primary response is likely to be mostly IgM, whereas antibody measured more than 2 weeks after a primary response, or any time after a secondary or subsequent response, is likely to be mostly IgG.

Although such tests are not typically available for bovine pathogens, if both agent-specific IgM and IgG can be measured in the same serum sample at the same time, the information supports the estimation of how recently the patient was infected or vaccinated. A patient with measurable serum IgM but no IgG against an agent was likely infected or vaccinated within the past 4 weeks, whereas a patient with both IgM and IgG was likely exposed within the past 4 to 8 weeks, and a patient with measurable IgG but not IgM was likely exposed more than 8 weeks ago (again, these times are approximate). Measurement of both IgM and IgG has been used to help differentiate recent infection from past infection or vaccination in horses with West Nile virus infection[4] and in people with severe acute respiratory syndrome coronavirus 2 (SARS-CoV-2) infection,[5] among other examples.

Specific Serologic Tests Commonly Used in Bovine Diagnostics

A variety of tests can be used to identify infectious agent-specific antibody in serum, with each test having benefits and drawbacks. At present, enzyme-linked immunosorbent assay (ELISA) and serum neutralizing (SN) (also known as virus neutralizing, VN) antibody tests are by far the most commonly used in veterinary diagnostic laboratories. Lateral flow assays, a type of ELISA, are often used for rapid patient-side identification of antigens or antibodies, but these are not currently readily available to identify agent-specific antibodies in cattle. Hemagglutination–inhibition (HI) assays are offered by many diagnostic laboratories for the detection of antibodies to influenza, but currently these are unlikely to be relevant for bovine diagnostics. In the United States, agar gel immunodiffusion (AGID) tests are occasionally used to identify agent-specific antibodies, most commonly in animals tested prior to export. The complement fixation (CF) test was historically required for some applications, but the test is relatively cumbersome and subject to error, thus it has largely been phased out. Indirect immunofluorescent antibody tests have also been used for serologic diagnostics, but these have largely been replaced by ELISA tests. Given the ubiquitous use of ELISA and the SN/VN assay, those two tests will be described in more detail here.

Table 1
Concentrations of coronavirus-specific antibody classes in serum of seronegative calves (*n* = 5) before exposure (Day 0) and weekly after oral and nasal exposure with live bovine coronavirus, as measured by ELISA[2]

Serum Coronavirus-Specific Antibody	Day 0	Day 7	Day 14	Day 21	Day 28	Day 35
IgM	neg	2.7	4.1	2.3	1.5	0.7
IgG1	neg	neg	3.2	4.3	4.5	5.1
IgG2	neg	neg	neg	1.4	1.8	2.1
IgA	neg	neg	1.6	2.2	2.7	2.7

Table 2
Pattern of serum bovine respiratory syncytial virus (BRSV)-specific antibody production after intramuscular vaccination of seronegative calves ($n = 5$) with modified-live virus, as measured by ELISA

Serum BRSV-Specific Antibody	Mean (Range) Day of First Detection	Mean (Range) Day of Peak Titer	Mean (Range) Peak Titer
IgM[a]	6 (6–6)	7.3 (6–8)	167 (20–320)
IgG1	16.8 (10–24)	31 (31–31)	2816 (1280–5120)
IgG2[b]	50.5 (31–70)	50.5 (31–70)	60 (40–80)
IgA	Not detected	Not detected	Not detected

[a] Excludes 2 nonresponding calves.
[b] Excludes 3 nonresponding calves.[3]

Characteristics of the enzyme-linked immunosorbent assay

ELISA assays can be designed to identify either antibodies or antigens (eg, microbes or their components) in bovine samples. In the context of serology, ELISAs are commonly used to detect agent-specific antibodies in serum, nasal secretions, or other fluids. For example, an ELISA can be used to detect serum, plasma, or milk antibodies to *Mycobacterium avium* ssp. paratuberculosis for Johne's disease diagnosis.[6] The steps of an ELISA to detect agent-specific antibodies in serum or other fluid are shown in **Fig. 2**. Note that an ELISA can be designed to detect antibodies of all classes (ie, total antibody) directed against an agent, or it can be designed to identify only IgG, or other classes or subclasses; the exact antibody identified will

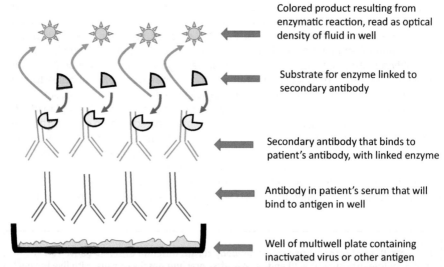

Colored product resulting from enzymatic reaction, read as optical density of fluid in well

Substrate for enzyme linked to secondary antibody

Secondary antibody that binds to patient's antibody, with linked enzyme

Antibody in patient's serum that will bind to antigen in well

Well of multiwell plate containing inactivated virus or other antigen

Fig. 2. Steps of an ELISA used to detect infectious agent-specific antibody in serum. Patient serum is added to wells of a mutiwell plate previously coated with antigen of interest, such as whole inactivated virus; serum is allowed to incubate. After washing, secondary antibody that will bind to patient antibody and which has been linked to an enzyme is added, and allowed to incubate. After washing, substrate for the enzyme is added, and allowed to react, forming a colored product that increases the optical density of the fluid in the well. The optical density is read by a spectrophotometer in a plate reader, with increasing optical density indicating higher concentration of specific antibody.

depend on the type of secondary antibody used. In diagnostic laboratories ELISAs used to measure agent-specific antibodies in serum will be likely be designed to measure IgG, or perhaps total bovine immunoglobulin. Competitive ELISAs can also be designed, which include a step in which a known amount of some other antibody to the agent in question is added to the reaction, and any antibody present in the serum sample being tested must "compete" for binding sites on the plate. In a competitive ELISA, a low signal means more antibody in the tested sample, because it will have "out competed" the antibody in the known positive sample included in the reaction. Competitive ELISAs can be characterized by particularly high assay sensitivity and specificity.

The ELISA has replaced many other serologic tests used historically because it is relatively simple to run, it is amenable to being automated, and it can be designed for high assay sensitivity and specificity. ELISA kits can be purchased for the detection of bovine antibodies to some infectious agents, meaning that all components of the ELISA are sold together, with instructions for each step. When kits are available, they can be relatively expensive, meaning that an in-house ELISA may be most cost-effective for the assay of a large number of samples. Designing an in-house test requires that all components of the ELISA must be purchased separately or created, and each step of the ELISA must be optimized. Whereas ELISA assays are widely used in bovine serologic diagnosis, it is not always easy or even possible to find a lab that runs an ELISA to measure antibodies to an uncommon agent, or to measure IgA or IgM against an agent. Some specialized equipment is also required to run a classic ELISA (eg, the plate reader), thus this version of the assay is not feasible for use in typical veterinary practices. However, modifications of the ELISA, such as the lateral flow assay, are certainly feasible for use in veterinary practice.

An ELISA may be designed to measure antibodies to whole infectious agents, or to only a single component of the agent. For example, ELISA has been used to measure bovine serum antibodies to whole *Mannheimia haemolytica* organisms, or to the leukotoxin secreted by *M. haemolytica*.[7] A source of purified leukotoxin would be necessary to create an *M haemolytica* leukotoxin-antibody-detecting ELISA; generating purified leukotoxin is beyond the scope of work done in most diagnostic laboratories. For this reason, ELISAs to specific components of an agent are usually used only by research laboratories. Similarly, ELISAs used to identify antibodies to viruses can be developed to measure antibodies against whole virions, or to viral components. For example, some commercially available ELISA kits for diagnosis of antibodies to bovine leukosis virus (BLV) detect antibodies to the viral envelope glycoprotein gp51.[8,9] Nonspecific reactions may be less troublesome in ELISAs designed to identify antibodies to components of agents.

The final result of an ELISA is a colored product; in the classic version of the assay, the colored product causes an increase in optical density (OD) of the fluid in the well of the microwell plate, measured by a spectrophotometer in a plate reader. Depending on how the ELISA is designed, the OD will either be directly related to the concentration of antibody in the sample (higher OD means more antibody), or the OD will be inversely related to the concentration of antibody (higher OD means less antibody). However, the OD alone can be difficult to interpret, so the laboratory reporting the result will need to establish and report cutoffs for positive or negative results, if these are not already defined by an ELISA kit being used. Because the OD is a continuous number, a "suspect" range may also be reported that is not clearly positive or negative. Determination of positive/negative cutoffs for test results requires analysis and interpretation that may not be simple; this concept is discussed more elsewhere in this issue.[10] Alternatively, the result for a sample can be reported as a ratio of sample

OD to that of a known positive (positive control) or known negative (negative control) standard tested in the same ELISA at the same time. However, the value the ratio of sample OD to positive or negative control that represents a positive or negative test result still needs to be determined and reported by the lab. Finally, ELISA results can be reported as a titer, a dilution at which the sample reaches the cutoff for a positive or negative test. So, for example, if a sample is tested at dilutions of 1:10, 1:100, and 1:1000, and the ELISA indicates presence of antibody in the 1:10 and 1:100 dilutions of the sample, but not the 1:1000 dilution, the sample would likely be reported to have a titer of 1:100, or perhaps simply 100. A veterinarian receiving results from ELISA testing for the first time may wish to discuss the significance of the results with a knowledgeable lab representative if the report is not clear.

It is important to note that the presence of agent-specific antibodies, as identified by ELISA testing of serum or other material, does not guarantee that the individual from which the sample was collected will be protected from infection or disease. The presence of antibody in an animal indicates that the animal has mounted a humoral immune response (unless the antibody was acquired passively). However, a humoral immune response is not always sufficient to prevent infection or disease. The protective significance of measurable antibodies to an agent depends on a variety of factors related to the host immune response, the virulence and infective dose of the agent, and the pathogenesis of disease caused by the agent.

Characteristics of the serum (virus) neutralizing (SN/VN) assay

The SN assay, also known as the VN assay, is an assay that quantifies antibody that prevents a specific virus from attaching to and infecting host cells. Thus, the SN assay is an assay that measures a specific immune function. In this context, "neutralization" means to prevent a virus from attaching to cells (thereby preventing infection). Thus, antibodies measured by SN assay provide more direct evidence of protective immunity than do antibodies measured by ELISA, which may not be neutralizing antibodies. However, an animal with measurable SN antibodies could still be vulnerable to infection or disease, based on several factors mentioned above. The steps of the SN assay are shown in **Fig. 3**. Because the SN assay requires the use of live virus and live cells susceptible to viral infection, it is technically more demanding than the ELISA, and not amenable for use outside diagnostic or research laboratories with approval to work with pure cultures of live bovine pathogens. Because live agents, even agents as simple as virions or individual cells, can behave in unpredictable or undesired ways, the SN assay is prone to certain types of error related to variability of the virus or cell stocks used for the assay. Also, because the final outcome measured is virus growth in cells, which may or may not occur, depending on the presence of neutralizing antibody in the sample tested, the SN assay takes at least a few days to complete, because time must pass to allow the possibility of virus growth. In contrast, any ELISA can be run in a few hours, with results potentially available the same day the assay is begun.

By definition, SN assays measure antibodies to viruses. Although it is possible to design an assay to measure antibodies that prevent bacteria from attaching to cells,[11] or to measure antibodies that block the action of bacterial toxins,[12] such assays are technically difficult and generally beyond the scope work in diagnostic laboratories, so assays to measure bacterial- or bacterial toxin-neutralizing antibodies are principally used only in research.

USE AND INTERPRETATION OF SEROLOGIC TESTING

Testing to measure infectious agent-specific antibodies is likely to be useful for three reasons:

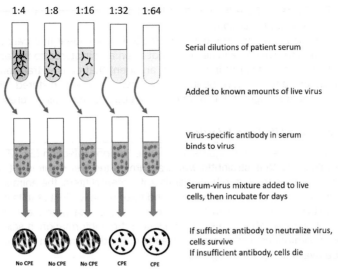

1:4   1:8   1:16   1:32   1:64

Serial dilutions of patient serum

Added to known amounts of live virus

Virus-specific antibody in serum binds to virus

Serum-virus mixture added to live cells, then incubate for days

If sufficient antibody to neutralize virus, cells survive
If insufficient antibody, cells die

No CPE   No CPE   No CPE   CPE   CPE

Fig. 3. Steps of a serum (virus) neutralizing assay. Dilutions of patient serum are added to known amounts of virus, allowed to incubate for a short time, then added to cultures of live cells susceptible to infection by the virus. Cells are allowed to incubate for days (the exact number of days depends on how fast the virus grows). Cell cultures are then read for cytopathic effect (CPE) due to viral infection, and the well treated with the highest dilution of serum that prevents cytopathic effect indicates the titer. In the example in the figure, the SN titer is 1:16.

1. To determine whether cattle have been infected with an agent in the past; or if they are currently infected with an agent that is difficult to identify by culture or polymerase chain reaction;
2. To determine whether cattle have developed antibodies in response to vaccination against specific agents; or,
3. To survey for evidence of infection by specific agents in populations of cattle.

As discussed above, it must be remembered that identification of antibodies to an infectious agent in an animal does not guarantee the animal will be protected from infection or disease. Moreover, antibody titers that are high enough to prevent disease may not prevent infection, meaning that an animal with antibodies may stay healthy if infected, but may still be susceptible to infection and subsequent transmission of infection to other in-contact animals. Also, antibody titers that may prevent disease in animals managed under good conditions may be inadequate to prevent disease in animals managed under conditions of poor biosecurity or biocontainment, inadequate nutrition, crowded conditions, or frequent mixing with animals from various sources.

Veterinarians or producers sometimes ask whether serology can be used to determine whether cattle are likely to be protected from disease without further vaccination. Given the number of variables that influence whether an animal with a certain antibody titer is likely to develop disease following exposure to an infectious agent, it is perhaps not surprising that it is hard to find reports of titers generally accepted to be protective against various diseases.

When serology is used to identify *evidence of past or current infection*, results must be interpreted considering whether:

1. Antibodies measured are the result of infection by an agent that causes life-long (persistent or latent) infection;
2. Antibodies measured are the result of infection by an agent that causes transient infection, and for which vaccines have not been administered to tested cattle;
3. Antibodies are the result of infection by an agent that causes transient infection, and for which vaccines have been, or may have been, administered, and
4. The animal is at an age at which maternal antibodies may still be present.

Agents that Cause Life-Long Infection

Interpretation of titers against agents that cause life-long infection (eg, *M. avium* ssp. paratuberculosis, BLV) is straightforward: assuming the test result is a true positive, and that the animal is too old to have persistent maternal titers, the animal is infected. (Estimating the likelihood of false positive and false negative test results is discussed elsewhere in this issue.[10]) The clinical significance of the measured titer must be determined based on research of the specific disease, from information in scientific publications or presentations. Unfortunately, clearly defined information regarding all risks may not be available for many agents.

Agents Causing Transient Infection, with no History of Vaccination

Interpretation of antibody titers in this situation is also relatively simple: assuming the test result is a true positive and maternal antibodies are unlikely, the presence of titers indicates past or possibly current infection. Whether infection occurred recently may be estimated based on how high titers are, but this can be difficult to interpret accurately. Relatively high titers can suggest recent infection, but relatively low titers may not rule out recent infection, especially if the infection was too recent to allow titers to become high, or if the animal used antibodies to fight off infection. What constitutes a high titer varies depending on the agent and type of assay used to measure the titer. Experienced diagnosticians may be willing to advise whether a given titer is relatively high; however, such expert opinion may not be definitive. Estimating the likelihood of past or recent infection is aided by testing multiple individuals in the group that may have been infected, because in any group, some cattle will have higher titers than others. Simultaneous measurement of IgM and IgG directed against the agent could help to more accurately estimate when infection occurred, but tests to measure both IgM and IgG directed against common bovine infectious agents seem to be rarely used. Paired serology, discussed below, can be helpful to determine more definitively whether the infection occurred recently.

Agents Causing Transient Infection, with History of Vaccination

Accurate interpretation of antibody titers in this situation can be difficult. Generally speaking, vaccination causes serum antibody titers to increase over a period of 4 to 8 weeks, after which antibody titers stay elevated for a period, and then decline. However, the exact length of time required for vaccine-induced antibodies to decline following vaccination, assuming no natural exposure, varies considerably depending on the agent, the type of vaccine administered, whether the vaccine includes an adjuvant, and the type of adjuvant in the vaccine. For example, a single dose of certain vaccines can induce serum antibody titers that can be measured for at least 140 days.[13,14] Moreover, if cattle have been vaccinated and then are naturally exposed repeatedly, such as can occur for commonly circulating endemic viruses (eg, bovine respiratory syncytial virus, BRSV), antibody titers may be periodically reboosted, so that animals may never become seronegative. As described above, an experienced diagnostician may be willing to estimate whether titers are "very high" and support recent infection or vaccination. However, given multiple sources of uncertainty, it is practically impossible to interpret the significance of single serum antibody titers to endemic agents against which cattle have also been vaccinated. Paired serology is necessary to determine whether infection recently occurred.

Serologic testing to confirm recent infection or vaccination against bacterial agents that are also commensal organisms, such as *M haemolytica* or *Escherichia coli,* can be particularly difficult to interpret, because seroconversion may result from normal commensal exposure. For example, calves have been shown to develop serum antibodies to *M haemolytica* and *Pasteurella multocida* in the absence of any evidence of disease.[7] The complexity of interpreting serologic responses to commensals that can also cause disease may be the reason that serologic tests for such agents have historically rarely been offered by many diagnostic laboratories.

Passively Acquired Antibodies

When interpreting serologic data, it is necessary to consider whether maternal antibodies were likely present in the cattle sampled. The half-lives of maternal antibodies to common respiratory viruses have been measured and determined to range from 13 to 28 days.[15,16] However, the exact time to seronegative status for a calf will depend on the maximum concentration of maternal antibodies present at the beginning of life, and also whether the calf had to use up antibodies to fight infection. Although the number of relevant variables make it impossible to state a single age at which maternal antibodies can be reliably presumed to be absent in a calf, a conservative estimate is that maternal antibodies are unlikely to be present in calves older than 8 months of age. Research has shown that a high proportion of recently weaned beef calves entering feedlots or stocker operations are seronegative to many common viruses.[17–19]

Negative feedback systems in the humoral immune response prevent serum antibodies from increasing infinitely.[20,21] In other words, once serum antibodies to a specific agent have reached a certain level, they do not normally increase further in response to vaccination or transient infection. *Therefore, vaccination or infection may not cause increased antibody titers in calves with moderate to high concentrations of maternal antibodies to the agent.*[22–25] For this reason it may be impossible to use serology to reliably identify recent infection, or to measure the response to vaccination, in calves with maternal antibodies, even if paired serology is used. In calves vaccinated in the face of maternal antibodies, other immune responses, such as cell-mediated immune responses, can occur even if serum antibodies do not increase,[26,27] although it is usually not practically possible for diagnostic laboratories to measure cell-mediated immune responses to specific agents. Possible outcomes of vaccination of calves with or without maternal antibodies are shown in **Fig. 4.** Similar responses can also be seen in individuals with actively acquired antibodies.

Paired Serology

Paired serology is the use of 2 serum samples collected from the same animal, separated by 2 to 4 weeks of time, to document a rising antibody titer, indicating an active humoral response due to recent infection or vaccination. When one wishes to determine whether cattle are infected with an agent, paired serology is easier to interpret than a single serum sample when cattle may have antibodies to the agent due to past infection or vaccination. To conduct paired serology, a serum sample is collected from one or more individuals at the time of vaccination or suspected infection (the "acute" sample), and a second sample is collected 2 to 4 weeks later (the "convalescent" sample). Both samples are then tested, and a fourfold increase in titer—or an

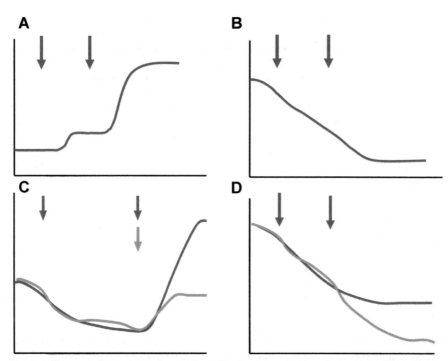

Fig. 4. Influence of serum agent-specific antibody concentration at the time of infection or vaccination on the subsequent serum antibody response. (*A*) In individuals with low serum concentrations of agent-specific antibody, the first exposure (*red arrow, left*) leads to a modest increase, and the second exposure (*red arrow, right*) leads to greater and more rapid increase. (*B*) In individuals with agent-specific antibody, specific antibody concentration may decrease, even after multiple exposures (*red arrows*).[25] (*C*) Serum antibody concentrations may continue to decline after the first exposure (*red arrow, left*). However, a second exposure (*red arrow, right*) after antibodies have disappeared may lead to an anamnestic-type response (*red line*), as compared with individuals not previously exposed (*blue line*).[22,23] (*D*) Serum agent-specific antibody concentrations may decline in spite of exposure (*red arrows*), but total serum antibody (*red line*) may stay higher longer than in unexposed individuals (*blue line*).[24,25]

increase of 2 dilutions—indicates "seroconversion": an active humoral response indicating a response to vaccination or infection. When serum titers are tested in a series of 1:2 dilutions, the possible titer will always be a multiple of 2: 1:2, 1:4, 1:8, etc. Seroconversion is indicated by a fourfold rise, which is the same as two dilutions. For example, if a calf has an acute titer of 1:16, and a convalescent titer of at least 1:64 (a fourfold increase, representing two dilutions), then that calf has seroconverted. If a calf has an acute titer of 1:16, and a convalescent titer of 1:32, it has not seroconverted as classically defined, even though the titer has apparently increased. This convention of using a fourfold dilution to indicate an active immune response is at least in part because a biological sample like serum, which contains many antimicrobial factors, is likely to demonstrate small amounts of day-to-day variation in antimicrobial activity that may not be due to specific antibodies. Note that if a fourfold *decrease* in titer is measured, this is also considered to indicate that the animal had a recent humoral response, but that the results of the response are being measured at a later time point in the response (**Fig. 5**). If paired serology is to be used, it is important to collect the

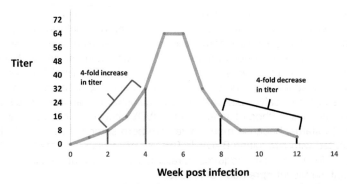

Fig. 5. Results of paired serology which indicate recent vaccination or infection. Fourfold increase or decrease in titer between two consecutive samples collected 2 to 4 weeks apart indicates active humoral immune response, with sampling having occurred either earlier (when titer is increasing) or later (when titer is decreasing) in the response. Note: although this figure indicates a rapid increase then decrease in antibody titer for convenient depiction of the principle, antibody titers can sometimes stay elevated for months before declining.

two samples no more than 4 weeks apart; a larger time interval may cause the relative change caused by increasing or decreasing antibody production to be missed, leading to an incorrect interpretation of the results. Similarly, sampling animals that were infected more than 2 to 4 weeks before the acute sample is collected may lead to false negative results in paired serologic testing, if seroconversion has already occurred when the first (acute) serum sample is collected.

When submitting samples for paired serology, the first serum sample should be separated from clotted blood and stored in a freezer at −20° C (−4° F) until the second sample is collected. *Then both samples should be submitted to the same diagnostic laboratory for testing at the same time, on the same day.* This is very important, because the ELISA and SN/VN tests are subject to day-to-day variation that can impact the titer measured, thus adding error to the interpretation of the results if the acute and convalescent samples are not tested on the same day. Interlaboratory agreement in results of serology has been shown to vary from good to only fair for different assays,[28] thus samples to be compared over time should always be submitted to the same laboratory.

The requirement that paired samples be tested together means that it takes a few weeks from the time the acute sample is collected to obtain the results of paired serology. Therefore, paired serology is not helpful for deciding how to manage disease at the time the disease is occurring, but it can provide clear evidence of infection that can be used to plan management (eg, vaccination strategies, or modified biocontainment or biosecurity practices) to prevent future outbreaks. When using paired serology to determine the cause of an outbreak in a group or herd, it is important to sample multiple animals, because not all animals in the group will be found to seroconvert at the same time. Information to guide sample size calculations is presented elsewhere in this issue.[29]

SEROLOGIC DIAGNOSIS FOR SURVEILLANCE

Serologic diagnosis can be used effectively for surveillance and eradication of certain diseases, as has been evident with brucellosis eradication programs in many countries.[30] A serum ELISA test is used as a component of the US voluntary bovine Johne's disease control program.[6] In addition to national control programs, serology can be used for surveillance for endemic diseases. For example, inclusion of unvaccinated seronegative sentinel animals in herds to identify herds with cattle persistently infected with BVDV (BVDV PI) has been attempted.[31,32] However, in one study, that approach only identified 53% of the herds with at least one BVDV PI animal.[32] It has been suggested that, at least in dairy herds, where the practice could be convenient, testing serum collected from calves before they nurse colostrum for antibodies to BVDV could be a more effective method of screening for BVDV circulation in herds than testing all calves for PI status, because more calves are born seropositive than are born PI in herds infected with circulating BVDV.[33] The use of serology to screen for the occurrence of endemic diseases requires careful planning so that vaccination schemes do not confuse the interpretation of results.

THE INFLUENCE OF TEST PERFORMANCE ON SEROLOGIC DIAGNOSIS

Implicit in this article is the concept that any test will at least occasionally produce false positive or false negative results. In other words: "Problems may arise if test results are uncritically considered as being the same as the unknown true value."[34] The impact of disease prevalence on test accuracy is particularly relevant to some clinical situations (eg, screening healthy animals), and this can be a truly difficult concept for a clinician to use well. A discussion of this topic is covered elsewhere in this issue[10] and in other sources.[34,35] Clinicians and diagnosticians should understand the impact of test performance in the populations of animals they test, at least for tests they use regularly, or in high-cost situations.

THE INFLUENCE OF SAMPLING HANDLING ON SEROLOGIC DIAGNOSIS

Sample handling practices of blood or other materials collected for serologic diagnosis can impact the quality and reliability of results. Sample collection and handling is discussed in more detail elsewhere in this issue.[36] In general, antibodies are somewhat stable over a range of moderate temperatures. Being at room temperature for 24 h, or being in a working refrigerator for several days, should not change antibody concentrations in a sample to a degree that is likely to change the test outcome. Antibodies are also tolerant of freeze-thaw cycles; a recent report indicated that up to 14 freeze-thaw cycles did not change the amount of SARS-CoV-2 antibody identified by ELISA in 11 human serum samples.[37] For long-term storage (weeks to years), samples containing antibodies for future assay should be kept at −20° C (−4° F). However, if serum is not pulled off clotted blood within 24 h, the serum sample may become hemolyzed, which could interfere with some serologic tests. Also, if the sample was not collected aseptically, bacterial proliferation in the sample may cause it to be unusable, particularly in SN tests that rely on exposure to live cells in culture that must be kept free from bacterial contamination. Before undertaking expensive serologic diagnosis, such as submission of samples from a large number of animals, confirm with the receiving diagnostic laboratory how samples should be collected, processed, and stored before and during shipment, to ensure the best possible outcome.

CLINICS CARE POINTS

- Serology is used to measure the amount of antigen-specific antibody in serum of cattle, to determine whether cattle have been infected with or vaccinated against a specific agent.

- Seroconversion, a 2-fold or greater increase in antibody titer between a sample collected during infection (acute), and a second sample collected 2 to 4 weeks later (convalescent), indicates recent infection or vaccination.
- Acute and convalescent samples should be submitted to the diagnostic laboratory at the same time, and tested on the same day, for accurate evaluation of seroconversion.
- Calves that still have circulating maternal antibodies may not seroconvert when they are vaccinated or infected; lack of seroconversion does not indicate that a calf has not been infected or immunized.

REFERENCES

1. Tizard I. Antibodies: Soluble Antigen Receptors. In: Veterinary Immunology. 10th edition. St. Louis: Elsevier; 2018. p. 162–72.
2. Heckert RA, Saif LJ, Mengel JP, et al. Isotype-specific antibody responses to bovine coronavirus structural proteins in serum, feces, and mucosal secretions from experimentally challenge-exposed colostrum-deprived calves. Am J Vet Res 1991;52:692–9.
3. Kimman TG, Westenbrink F, Schreuder BEC, et al. Local and systemic antibody response to bovine respiratory syncytial virus infection and reinfection in calves with and without maternal antibodies. J Clin Microbiol 1987;25:1097–106.
4. Ostlund EN, Crom RL, Pedersen DD, et al. Equine West Nile encephalitis, United States. Emerg Infect Dis 2001;7:665–9.
5. Suhandynata RT, Hoffman MA, Kelner MJ, et al. Longitudinal monitoring of SARS-CoV-2 IgM and IgG seropositivity to detect COVID-19. J Appl Lab Med 2020;5:908–20.
6. USDA APHIS. Uniform Program Standards for the Voluntary Bovine Johne's Disease Control Program. 2010. Available at: https://www.aphis.usda.gov/animal_health/animal_diseases/johnes/downloads/johnes-ups.pdf. Accessed July 29, 2022.
7. Prado ME, Prado TM, Payton M, et al. Maternally and naturally acquired antibodies to *Mannheimia haemolytica* and *Pasteurella multocida* in beef calves. Vet Immunol Immunopathol 2006;111:301–7.
8. Zooetis. Enzootic Bovine Leukosis. 2022. Available at: https://diagnostics.zoetis.com/species/ruminant/enzootic-bovine-leukosis/enzootic-bovine-leukosis.aspx. Accessed July 31, 2022.
9. Bioscience Indical. Svanovir BLV gp51-Ab (2 ELISA plates). 2022. Available at: https://shop.indical.com/en/assays-and-reagents/svanovir-blv-gp51-ab-2-elisa-plates.html. Accessed July 28, 2022.
10. Buczinski S. Interpretation and analysis of diagnostic tests and performance. Vet Clin Food Anim 2022. In press.
11. Yokoyama H, Peralta RC, Diaz R, et al. Passive protective effect of chicken egg yolk immunoglobulins against experimental enterotoxigenic *Escherichia coli* infection in neonatal piglets. Infect Immun 1992;60:998–1007.
12. Hodgins DC, Shewin PE. Serologic responses of young colostrum fed dairy calves to antigens of *Pasteurella haemolytica* A1. Vaccine 1998;20:2018–25.
13. Fulton RW, Burge LJ, O'ffay JM, et al. Serum antibody response in calves receiving modified live and/or inactivated vaccines containing bovine herpesvirus-1, bovine viral diarrhea virus, parainfluenza-3 virus, and bovine respiratory syncytial virus immunogens. Bov Pract 1997;31(2):90–6.

14. Fulton RF, Burge LJ. Bovine viral diarrhea virus types 1 and 2 antibody response in calves receiving modified live virus or inactivated vacines. Vaccine 2001;19: 264–74.

15. Kirkpatrick J, Fulton RW, Burge LJ, et al. Passively transferred immunity in newborn calves, rates of antibody decay, and effect on subsequent vaccination with modified live virius vaccine. Bov Pract 2001;35:47–55.

16. Mechor GD, Virtala AMK, Dubovi EJ, et al. The half-life for maternally derived immunoglobulin G anti-viral antibodies in data from an observational field study. Bov Pract 2001;35:131–6.

17. Fulton RW, Purdy CW, Confer AW, et al. Bovine viral diarrhea viral infections in feeder calves with respiratory disease: interactions with *Pasteurella* spp., parainfluenza-3 virus, and bovine respiratory syncytial virus. Can J Vet Res 2000;64:151–9.

18. Richeson JT, Beck PA, Gadberry MS, et al. Effects of on-arrival versus delayed modified live virus vaccination on health, performance,and serum infectious bovine rhinotracheitis titers of newly received beef calves. J Anim Sci 2008;86: 999–1005.

19. Griffin CM, Scott JA, Karisch BB, et al. A randomized controlled trial to test the effect of on-arrival vaccination and deworming on stocker cattle health and growth performance. Bov Pract 2018;52:26–33.

20. Heyman B. Regulation of antibody responses via antibodies, complement, and Fc receptors. Annu Rev Immunol 2000;18:709–37.

21. Arulraj T, Binder SC, Robert PA, et al. Synchronous germinal center onset impacts the efficiency of antibody responses. Front Immunol 2019. https://doi.org/10. 3389/fimmu.2019.02116.

22. Brar JS, Johnson DW, Muscoplat CC, et al. Maternal immunity to infectious bovine rhinotracheitis virus and bovine virus diarrhea viruses: duration and effect on vaccination in young calves. Am J Vet Res 1978;39:241–4.

23. Menanteau-Horta AM, Ames TR, Johnsonn DW, et al. Effect of maternal antibody upon vaccination with infectious bovine rhinotracheitis and bovine virus diarrhea vaccines. Can J Comp Med 1985;49:10–4.

24. Van Donkersgoed J, Guenther C, Evans BN, et al. Effects of various vaccination protocols on passive and active immunity to *Pasteurella haemolytica* and *Haemophilus somnus* in beef calves. Can Vet J 1995;36:424–9.

25. Kaeberle M, Sealock R, Honeyman M. Antibody responses of young calves to inactivated viral vaccines. Proc Am Assoc Bov Pract 1998;31:229–32.

26. Ellis JA, Hassard LE, Cortese VS, et al. Effects of perinatal vaccination on humoral and cellular immune responses in cows and young calves. J Am Vet Med Assoc 1996;208:393–400.

27. Endsley JJ, Ridpath JF, Neill JD, et al. Induction of T lymphocytes specific for bovine viral diarrhea virus in calves with maternal antibody. Viral Immunol 2004;17:13–23.

28. Fang F, Collins-Emerson JM, Heuer C, et al. Interlaboratory and between-specimen comparisons of diagnostic tests for leptospirosis in cattle. J Vet Diagn Invest 2014;26:734–47.

29. Parker EM. Diagnostic strategies for populations. Vet Clin Food Anim 2022. In press.

30. Zhang N, Huang D, Wu W, et al. Animal brucellosis control or eradication programs worldwide: a systematic review of experiences and lessons learned. Prev Vet Med 2018;160:105–15.

31. Corbett EM, Grooms DL, Bolin SR, et al. Use of sentinel serology in a bovine viral diarrhea virus eradication program. J Vet Diagn Invest 2011;23:511–5.

32. Waldner CL, Campbell JR. Use of serologic evaluation for antibodies against bovine viral diarrhea virus for detection of persistently infected calves in beef herds. Am J Vet Res 2005;66:825–34.

33. Newcomer BW, Givens D. Diagnosis and control of viral diseases of reproductive importance, infectious bovine rhinotracheitis and bovine viral diarrhea. Vet Clin Food Anim 2016;32:425–41.

34. Hahn A, Podbielski A, Meyer T, et al. On detection thresholds-a review on diagnostic approaches in the infectious disease laboratory and the interpretation of their results. Acta Tropica 2020;105377.

35. Smith DR. Epidemioloigc tools for biosecurity and biocontainment. Vet Clin Food Anim 2002;18:157–75.

36. Monday JD. Maximizing value for diagnostic submissions. Vet Clin Food Anim 2022. In press.

37. Shurrab FM, Al-Sadeq DW, Amanullah F, et al. Effect of multiple freeze-thaw cycles on the detection of anti-SARS-CoV-2 IgG antibodies. J Med Microbiol 2021; 70:001402.

Toxicology and Analytical Chemistry

Christina Wilson-Frank, MS, PhD

KEYWORDS

- Diagnostic toxicology • Ruminant • Veterinary • Toxicology • Diagnostic testing
- Large animal

KEY POINTS

- Toxicoses in ruminant animals can result in significant economic losses to livestock owners/producers and pose a herd/flock health hazard to the remaining unaffected animals.
- Effective use of veterinary, toxicology/analytical chemistry laboratories is important when navigating toxicology cases in ruminants.
- Obtaining a complete case history and knowing what samples to collect and submit for toxicology testing will maximize the likelihood of diagnosis.

INTRODUCTION

Veterinary toxicology laboratories combine the use of clinical toxicology and analytical chemistry to investigate and diagnose poisoning intoxication cases in animals. They often provide toxicology testing services at the state, regional, and federal levels to clientele which can include veterinarians, veterinary pathologists, producers, animal owners, law enforcement, and government and state agencies. Veterinary toxicology laboratories have staff with expertise in veterinary, clinical toxicology, and also analytical chemistry. Often, the veterinary toxicologist consults with clients and coordinates information obtained from case histories to determine the appropriate analytical tests that should be performed for each case. After the toxicology tests are completed, the veterinary toxicologist interprets the results for the client. The specific toxicology tests provided by these laboratories can vary slightly depending on the laboratory's analytical capabilities. Although there is no "toxicology screen" or "poison screen" that can be performed as a single test on a diagnostic sample to detect all toxicants, toxins, and drugs, it is important to note that advances in analytical instrumentation have enabled toxicology/analytical chemistry laboratories to provide improved screening-

Indiana Animal Disease Diagnostic Laboratory, Department of Comparative Pathobiology, Purdue University College of Veterinary Medicine, 406 South University, West Lafayette, IN 47907-2065, USA
E-mail address: wilsonc@purdue.edu

Vet Clin Food Anim 39 (2023) 157–164
https://doi.org/10.1016/j.cvfa.2022.11.001
0749-0720/23/© 2022 Elsevier Inc. All rights reserved.

vetfood.theclinics.com

types of analyses to the veterinary community. For example, introduction of inductively coupled plasma with optical emission spectrometry (ICP/OES) or mass spectrometry (ICP/MS) has enabled toxicology laboratories to perform trace nutrient/heavy metal screens on environmental and biological samples. These new technologies permit the analysis of multiple trace nutrients or heavy metals with the additional benefit of smaller sample size minimum requirements.[1] Advances in gas chromatography, high-performance liquid chromatography, and ultra-high-performance liquid chromatography, have enabled toxicology laboratories to screen samples for a diverse range of analytes including but not limited to biotoxins, chemical toxicants, feed additives, vitamins A and E, and drugs or medications when combined with a variety of detectors.[2,3] Other analyses can also be performed that do not require instrumentation. This can include, but is not limited to; using colorimetric tests (eg, nitrate or cyanide testing), pH measurement (eg, testing for rumen acidosis), and gross observation or microscopic evaluation of rumen contents or gastrointestinal contents (eg, identification of poisonous plants material or seeds or foreign material). Regardless of the tests performed, there are instances in which toxicology/analytical chemistry laboratories are not able to provide a definitive diagnosis for a case. Limitations are often due to lack of a complete case history and/or inadequate sample type, amount, or quality. Therefore, this article is intended to provide some guidance with respect to the effective use of veterinary toxicology/analytical chemistry laboratories when navigating suspect primary toxicology cases in ruminants.

Case History

Partnering with the veterinary toxicology diagnostic specialists by providing a complete case history is essential when navigating suspect toxicoses in ruminants. This typically happens at the onset of the case; however, sometimes it can evolve subsequent to diagnostic testing, necropsy findings, and histopathology. There are instances in veterinary toxicology when the only clinical sign is that the animals were found dead, with minimal to no case history that can be provided. When taking a case history, minimal initial information to obtain includes documenting the species, breed, age(s), total number of animals in the group, if any medications were given, management risk activities before clinical presentation (eg, transport, processing, feed change, environment change), number of animals that are dead or showing clinical signs, and what clinical signs or behavior abnormalities were observed if witnessed. If multiple animals are affected, it suggests a common source of toxicity. The next important steps are to note the clinical signs observed, establish a timeline of exposure, and inquire about the environment to identify potential sources of exposure. When developing a list of differential diagnoses, the observed clinical signs are helpful in determining what types of toxins or toxicants should be included in that list. For example, are the animals showing signs of nervous system stimulation/depression, having gastrointestinal issues (eg, diarrhea), reproductive issues, showing exercise intolerance, or having difficulty standing or breathing? There can be instances in which ruminants can be exposed to a poison or chemical, but may not show clinical signs. If a known exposure is identified, testing should be conducted to ensure those being used as food animals do not have any actionable subclinical levels of that toxicant in biological samples, including milk, before being sold for human consumption. Information garnered from performing clinical chemistries can also help triage what groups of toxicants should be considered. For example, if the ruminant animal has significantly elevated liver enzymes, or notably increased blood urea nitrogen (BUN)/creatinine, or clinically significant increases in creatine kinase, then hepatotoxicants, or nephrotoxicants, or skeletal muscle toxicants, respectively would be ones to consider on the differential list. Establishing a timeline of exposure is important and includes inquiring about the earliest timeframe when the animal(s) appeared normal and comparing that with the timeframe in which clinical signs were observed or death occurred. This can be challenging because ruminants may be permitted to roam large areas and accuracy can depend on the opportunity and ability of the owner/producer to notice abnormalities. Whether animals are in a confined setting or permitted to roam, they often share a common environment and have access to the same water sources, pasture, and feedstuffs. Correlating recent changes in any of these factors, within proximity of the onset of clinical signs should be noted. Knowing what type of feedstuff or supplements are being given (feed, hay, silage, pasture forage, access to mineral blocks), if there are any plants in the pasture (particularly poisonous plants) or changes in the pasture quality are important. Assessment of water sources such as streams or ponds, access to any containers or bags of pesticide, waste piles, old equipment, abandoned buildings, oil derricks, or other source material should be noted. Interestingly, having an idea of the weather conditions before or during the onset of clinical signs can be significant. There are instances in which strong winds may blow down branches from cherry trees in the pasture or blow harmful blue–green algae to one concentrated area in a pond. When heavy rains occur, it is possible to have pesticide runoff to the extent that animals can be exposed if drinking from sources on property where the pesticides have been collected. When livestock are involved, there can be several affected, which can result in significant economic losses to livestock owners/producers and pose a herd/flock health hazard to the remaining unaffected animals. Therefore, the key to protecting the health of the remaining animals and to mitigate losses begins with obtaining a complete case history and also knowing what samples to collect and submit for toxicology testing.

Sample Submission

Environmental samples and feedstuffs

Ruminants often share the same environment and food sources. Therefore, it is not surprising that in most toxicology cases, the water source, pasture, forage, feedstuffs, or other source materials in the environment are often associated with toxicoses in ruminants. The common types of feedstuffs and environmental samples, including the minimum recommended volume/weights to collect, are listed in **Table 1**. Water sources to collect can include water in troughs or other areas on property for which animals have free access. This should include water from streams or ponds or areas of stagnant water on property. Plants growing in the same environment as the ruminant animals (eg, pasture) can be collected for plant identification and/or toxin testing. Collecting the whole plant, including roots, flowers, and seeds is encouraged. When collecting feed, silage, or hay samples, it is important to collect a representative sample of the feedstuff. There can be "hot spots" or areas in the feedstuff in which the toxicant is more concentrated. Mycotoxins, sources of botulism, blister beetles, and nitrates are frequently associated with "hot spot" issues in feedstuffs. Therefore, it is important to collect a sample that best represents the whole batch of feed or silage or bale of hay. Collecting hay is best done by trying to take core samples from the whole bale. Source material on property to collect can include mineral supplements/mixes, suspicious material on premises, or other unknown substances. If the sample is limited, it is best to collect all of the source material. When the feed or mineral supplement is implicated as a potential source of toxicity, the product details are important to note, especially in cases when there could be a manufacturing error. If an issue with a manufactured feed or mineral supplement is suspected, it is important to obtain, at minimum, the following information from the product:

	Minimum Recommended	
Sample	**Volume/Weight**	**Potential Toxicology Tests**
Water	2 liters	Blue–green algae toxins[a], heavy metals, nitrate, pesticides, sulfate, and urea
Plants	Whole plant	Plant/seed identification and plant toxin testing[b]
Silage/haylage Hay/grass	2 lbs (representative)	Botulism (hay), feed microscopy[c], ergot/fescue alkaloids, nitrate, and mycotoxins
Feed	2 lbs (representative)	Drugs/medications, ergot/fescue alkaloids, feed additives, feed microscopy, gossypol, heavy metals, ionophores, mycotoxins, sodium (salt), sulfate, trace minerals, urea, and Vitamin A, Vitamin E
Source material	All of suspect source	Variable (depending on case history and clinical signs)

Table 1
Environmental samples and feedstuffs

[a] Blue–green algae toxins: Additional collection should include mixing one volume of the water source with an equal volume of 10% neutral-buffered formalin (1:1) for algae identification.
[b] If cyanide testing is warranted, freeze plant immediately and ship frozen as freeze-thawing can volatilize the cyanide and compromise testing.
[c] Feed microscopy in silage/haylage/hay/grass samples can include blister beetle identification.

- Name of the product and product description that is on the label
- Type of container (eg, bag and block)
- Lot number and expiration date
- UPC code
- Purchase date and where it was purchased
- When the product was introduced to the animals

An important resource that is available to livestock owners/producers and the veterinary community is provided by the Food and Drug Administration Center for Veterinary Medicine (FDA CVM). If a problem is suspected with a manufactured feed or mineral supplement, an adverse event can be reported through the safety reporting portal at https://www.fda.gov/animal-veterinary/report-problem/reporting-problems-horse-or-other-livestock-feedfood. The FDA CVM reviews the information reported and, subsequent to diagnostic testing and investigations, they can initiate possible regulatory actions if warranted.

Biological samples
Veterinary toxicology/analytical chemistry laboratories analyze a variety of antemortem and postmortem samples for most toxicants of concern in ruminants. Analyzing these samples can reveal what the animal was exposed to and can indicate if the amount of toxicant present is diagnostic. There are a few limitations to testing biological samples from ruminant animals. One limitation is that there are some plant toxins and mycotoxins that are not detectable in biological samples and testing is limited to analyzing only environmental samples or feedstuffs. In addition, scenarios exist in which the timeframe between the onset of clinical signs and exposure to the toxicant can be several days to weeks. Depending on the half-life of the toxicant and the type to toxicant for which the animals were exposed, detecting the toxicant in biological samples may be challenging. In these instances, case history and availability of suspect environmental samples/feedstuffs becomes more important.

Antemortem samples. Testing antemortem samples can provide useful information from live animals, especially when samples are collected from ruminants currently experiencing clinical signs. Antemortem samples for toxicology analyses include; liver biopsies, whole blood, feces, serum/plasma, hair, milk, and urine. The minimum recommended sample volumes and weights for toxicology testing commonly used on antemortem sample are listed in **Table 2**. As a rule of thumb, the more sample you collect and send, the better. Toxicology testing in tissue biopsies is largely limited to the liver. Testing liver biopsies can be rewarding, particularly when there are concerns about heavy metal toxicities or trace mineral deficiencies. Other toxicology tests, such as vitamin A or E analyses, are limited to postmortem liver samples as they require a larger sample weight. Submitting liver biopsies for trace mineral analyses can also be useful when there are concerns about the nutritional status in the herd/flock. The minimum recommended sample weight for a liver biopsy is approximately 0.1 g. Depending on the type of biopsy needle used, multiple biopsies may need to be performed to meet this minimum weight. For example, a Stryker double-action, biopsy clamp (5.0 mm diameter) can obtain a biopsy sample of approximately 0.1 to 0.2 grams in size. Therefore, only one biopsy is needed. However, if using a Tru-cut biopsy needled, 0.025 grams is the maximum biopsy size that can be harvested. Therefore, approximately 4 biopsies are required. Liver biopsies should be collected in a sterile container (eg, red top tube) without saline or any other preservative and stored frozen or chilled until analysis. Whole blood should be collected in a blood collection tube containing an anticoagulant, preferably EDTA. If blood is permitted to clot, this will interfere with the toxicology laboratory's ability to aliquot (pipet) a homogeneous sample for analysis, which can compromise accurate quantitation of the toxicant of interest. Whole blood samples should be stored frozen or chilled before analysis. When whole blood samples are collected, with the intent of isolating serum/plasma for testing, measures should be taken to prevent hemolysis. Animals should be appropriately restrained, and samples collected with a large gauge needle, preferably with a vacuum needle system instead of with a syringe. Using small gauge needles to pull blood samples can sheer red blood cells on drawing. Avoid storing whole blood frozen before centrifuging and aliquotting the serum/plasma. Freezing and thawing whole blood will cause the red blood cells to lyse. Hemolysis can artificially decrease vitamin E levels in the sample and can also effect accurate quantitation of trace minerals. Although zinc deficiency or toxicity is not a common concern in ruminants, it is important to note that blood collection tubes with rubber stoppers contain considerable amounts of zinc.[4] Therefore, if zinc testing is requested, ensuring minimal contact of the blood sample with the rubber stopper will ensure accurate quantitation of zinc in the serum/plasma. Centrifuging the blood sample and removing the serum/plasma soon after collection of blood is best. Serum/plasma, milk, and urine samples should be frozen or chilled before analysis.

Postmortem samples. Necropsies are an essential diagnostic tool to use in the case of mortalities due to suspected toxicoses. Many of these cases benefit from information obtained by necropsies performed by trained veterinary pathologists, often available at a veterinary diagnostic laboratory. The gross findings or histopathological results are very rewarding when trying to deduce the nature of the toxicosis in diagnostic cases. Veterinary toxicology/analytical chemistry laboratories frequently rely on pathological or histopathological findings to guide what toxicology tests should be performed. A necropsy will also permit collecting more of a variety of biological samples, which broadens the scope of potential toxicology tests that can be performed to rule in or out differential diagnoses. This is why it is important to encourage

Table 2
Antemortem samples

Sample	Minimum Recommended Volume/Weight	Potential Toxicology Tests
Biopsy (liver)	0.1 g	Heavy metals and trace nutrients
Whole blood	2 mL (in EDTA)	Acetylcholinesterase activity and cyanide[a], Drugs/medications, heavy metals, trace nutrients, pesticides, and rodenticides
Feces	10 g	Botulism
Serum/plasma	5 mL	Ammonia, anatoxin-a, botulism, cantharidin, drugs/medications, ionophores, nitrate, pesticides, rodenticides, trace nutrients, Vitamin A, and Vitamin E
Hair	Collect such that sample measures $3/4$ inch when bunched together	Growth promotants
Milk	20 mL	Aflatoxin, antibiotics, pesticides, and heavy metals (lead)
Urine	50 mL	Ammonia, anatoxin-a, cantharidin, drugs/medications, and plant toxins

[a] Whole blood submitted for cyanide testing must be stored frozen immediately after collection.

clients to have a necropsy performed on any deceased animals as a full, diagnostic work-up will provide the best diagnostic information for the case. The minimum, recommended postmortem sample volumes and weights, including common toxicology tests for each, are listed in **Table 3**. If a toxicoses is suspected, but the case history is lacking or pathology is unremarkable or nonspecific, it is important to collect each sample listed in **Table 3** to cover all potential testing. The exception would be milk, which is obviously limited to a lactating animal. Of the samples listed, urine may be the most difficult sample to obtain from a deceased animal. At necropsy, the bladder is often empty, making it difficult to obtain the volume of urine needed for testing. Although not a traditional toxicology test, whole femurs can be submitted to assess the percentage of fat present in bone marrow. Some toxicology laboratories measure percent fat in bone marrow from femurs to support a postmortem diagnosis of starvation or malnutrition in cases of animal cruelty or neglect.[5] The results of this test are used in combination with body condition scores determined by the pathologist. When collecting rumen contents, it is important to try to collect as representative of a sample as possible. Be sure to collect any intact plant material, seeds, or foreign material that is observed on gross examination. All of the samples listed in **Table 3** should be stored frozen until analysis.

Veterinary Toxicology/Analytical Chemistry Laboratories

This article provides recommendations on the sample types and minimum sample volumes/weights to collect as well as the common, requested toxicology tests for each. Although most veterinary toxicology/analytical chemistry laboratories have common analytical capabilities, some may vary with regard to the preferred samples for testing, as well as the tests they offer to clients. Also, some laboratories have veterinary toxicologists and technical staff with expertise in a specific discipline of veterinary toxicology or are the experts with regard to a certain toxicant or group of toxicants.

Table 3
Postmortem samples

Sample	Minimum Recommended Volume/Weight	Potential Toxicology Tests
Bone	Whole rib bone or femur	Bone density, calcium, and phosphorus
Bone marrow	Whole femur	Percent fat
Brain	½ of brain	Acetylcholinesterase and sodium (salt)
CSF	1 mL	Sodium (salt) and magnesium
Gastrointestinal contents[a]	200 g	Ammonia, blue–green algae toxins, botulism, cantharidin, gossypol, heavy metals, ionophores, plant/seed identification, pH, plant toxins, pesticides, and rodenticides
Hair	Collect such that sample measures ¾ inch when bunched together	Growth promotants
Kidney	10 g	Drugs/medications, heavy metals,
Liver	20 g	Drugs/Medications, heavy metals, pesticides, plant toxins, rodenticides, sulfur, trace nutrients, Vitamin A, and Vitamin E
Milk	20 mL	Aflatoxin, antibiotics, pesticides, and heavy metals (lead)
Ocular fluid	1 mL (whole eyeball)	Ammonia, magnesium, and sodium
Retinal tissue	Whole eyeball	Growth promotants
Urine	50 mL	Anatoxin-a, cantharidin, drugs/medications, and plant toxins

[a] Gastrointestinal contents include rumen contents or intestinal contents.

Therefore, it is important to investigate which diagnostic laboratory has a toxicology/analytical chemistry laboratory that can provide the service needed for these cases in ruminants. To date, there are approximately 19 veterinary diagnostic laboratories in North America with toxicology/analytical chemistry sections. These laboratories are accredited by the American Association of Veterinary Laboratory Diagnosticians (AAVLD). A list of these laboratories can be found at https://www.aavld.org/accredited-labs.

SUMMARY

Veterinary toxicology laboratories use clinical toxicology and analytical chemistry to investigate and diagnose poisoning cases in animals. When ruminant animals are exposed to toxicants, it can lead to significant losses in the herd/flock and can pose a health hazard risk to remaining, unaffected animals on the premises. Therefore, knowing how to effectively use veterinary toxicology/analytical chemistry laboratories and how to approach each case during the investigatory and diagnostic process will help maximize the likelihood of diagnosis.

CLINICS CARE POINTS

- Toxicoses in ruminant animals can result in significant economic losses to livestock owners/producers and pose a herd/flock health hazard to the remaining unaffected animals.
- Effective use of veterinary, toxicology/analytical chemistry laboratories is important when navigating toxicology cases in ruminants.
- Obtaining a complete case history and knowing what samples to collect and submit for toxicology testing will maximize the likelihood of diagnosis.

DISCLOSURE

This author has nothing to disclose.

REFERENCES

1. Goulle JP, Saussereau E, Mahieu L, et al. Current role of ICP-MS in clinical toxicology and forensic toxicology: a metallic profile. Bioanal 2014;6(17):2245–59.
2. Mbughuni MM, Jannetto PJ, Langman LJ. Mass spectrometry applications for toxicology. J Internat Fed Clin Chem Lab Med 2016;27(4):272–87.
3. Viette V, Fathi M, Rudaz S, et al. Current role of liquid chromatography coupled to mass spectrometry in clinical toxicology screening methods. Clin Chem Lab Med 2011;49(7):1091–103.
4. Ralstin JO, Schnieder PJ, Blackstone L, et al. Serum zinc concentrations: contamination from laboratory equipment. J Parenter Enteral Nutr 1979;3(3):179–81.
5. Meyerholtz KA, Wilson CR, Everson RJ, et al. Quantitative assessment of the percent fat in domestic animal bone marrow. J Forensic Sci 2011;56:775–7.

Next-Generation Diagnostics for Pathogens

Rebecca P. Wilkes, DVM, PhD, DACVM (virology and bacteriology/mycology)

KEYWORDS

- Ruminant molecular diagnostics • Targeted NGS
- Next-generation sequencing pathogen detection • NGS infectious diseases

KEY POINTS

- Next-generation sequencing (NGS) is the latest molecular technology to be introduced into diagnostic laboratories.
- There are different ways to use the technology for pathogen detection and characterization, and the cost varies depending on the method used. The most cost-effective NGS method to detect pathogens in a clinical sample is targeted NGS.
- Targeted NGS includes a step to concentrate the sequences of pathogens present in the sample before sequencing, reducing the number of sequences needed to detect the pathogen. This step not only reduces cost but also limits detection to only those pathogens that are specifically targeted by the assay.
- This method is ideal for syndromic testing for ruminant diseases, such as calf scours and bovine respiratory disease complex, due to its ability to detect and characterize a wide range of pathogens (including bacteria, viruses, and parasites) with a single test.

INTRODUCTION

DNA sequencing has been around since the 1970s and was almost exclusively performed by the Sanger method (first-generation sequencing) until the early 2000s when the next generation of sequencing was created.[1,2] The Sanger method is still used extensively in animal infectious disease diagnostics, but it only allows for producing a single sequence up to 1000 base pairs in length. This method was used initially for the Human Genome Project, but due to its scaling limitations, the project costs billions of dollars and took 13 years to complete.[2] Unlike Sanger sequencing, next-generation sequencing (NGS) is massively parallel sequencing (simultaneous production of millions of sequences) and has the potential to sequence everything in a sample. To put this revolutionary advancement in sequencing into perspective NGS has reduced the cost of sequencing a human genome to $600,[3] and it now

Department of Comparative Pathobiology and Molecular Section Head, Animal Disease Diagnostic Laboratory, Purdue University College of Veterinary Medicine, 406 South University St., West Lafayette, IN 47907-2065, USA
E-mail address: rwilkes@purdue.edu

Vet Clin Food Anim 39 (2023) 165–173
https://doi.org/10.1016/j.cvfa.2022.09.003
0749-0720/23/© 2022 Elsevier Inc. All rights reserved.
vetfood.theclinics.com

only takes 1 to 2 days to obtain the full sequence. For a review of currently available sequencing technologies, including first-, second-, and third-generation technologies, see Slatko and colleagues.[4] NGS encompasses several different approaches (**Box 1**) that are discussed, with specific attention to targeted NGS (tNGS), which the author's group has found to be the most plausible of the approaches to incorporate into the veterinary diagnostic laboratory for detection of infectious diseases.

DISCUSSION
Next-Generation Sequencing Approaches and Incorporation into the Diagnostic Laboratory

Sequencing of a genome using NGS is referred to as whole genome sequencing (WGS). Based on the definition from US Food and Drug Administration (FDA), "whole genome sequencing reveals the complete DNA make-up of an organism, enabling us to better understand variations both within and between species."[5] WGS of human genomes has allowed huge advances in the area of neoplasia detection and individualized targeted treatment (personalized medicine), based on genetic characterization of tumors,[6] and additionally has advanced understanding of rare genetic diseases that previously could not be well studied without this technology. In veterinary medicine, WGS of animal genomes has provided insight into genetic diseases of animals,[7] and in production medicine, WGS is helping evaluation of genetic profiles with improved phenotypic traits, such as heritability associated with milk fat percentage and crude milk protein that could improve farm profitability.[8] The use of NGS for genomics is clear; however, how can this technology be used for infectious diseases?

WGS moved into the public health laboratories in the 2010s as a means of sequencing whole bacterial genomes to characterize these pathogens associated with outbreaks.[2] WGS is highly useful for outbreak detection due to its ability to provide a large amount of information from isolates such as species, strain type, and the presence of antibiotic resistance and virulence genes. Small differences between isolates (such as single nucleotide changes or polymorphisms) can be detected with WGS to easily identify highly similar or even identical isolates, which aids identification of outbreak source and ability to track spread.[2] WGS has also been introduced into the veterinary diagnostic laboratory as a means of identifying bacterial resistance genes from isolates from veterinary patients through programs with the United States Department of Agriculture[9] and FDA[10] as part of The National Action Plan for Combating Antibiotic-Resistant bacteria (CARB). Although a molecular method, WGS tends to be limited to isolates for bacterial pathogens and is not generally performed directly from the clinical sample, unlike polymerase chain reaction (PCR). Also, although WGS as an NGS approach is valuable for outbreak tracing or characterizing isolates, its use for individual patient diagnostics is less clear.[2,11]

Box 1
Next-generation sequencing approaches

WGS: is sequencing the complete DNA or RNA make-up of an individual organism and is generally performed for clinical isolates.

mNGS: also referred to as deep or shotgun sequencing, is an NGS approach in which all genomic content (DNA and/or RNA) of a clinical or environmental sample is sequenced.

tNGS: use of capture probes or PCR to increase amount of pathogen before sequencing; improves sensitivity of pathogen detection but limits which pathogens are detected.

mNGS, metagenomic NGS; tNGS, targeted NGS; WGS, whole genome sequencing.

Another advantage of NGS is that there is no need to know what pathogens are present in the sample to detect them (hypothesis-free diagnostic method); there is no requirement for pathogen-specific primers with this method. This advantage allows for discovery of previously unrecognized organisms; it also allows for detection of variants that may have been missed with older primers, because viruses tend to change over time. Use of NGS in this manner is called metagenomic NGS (mNGS), also referred to as deep or shotgun sequencing, in which all genomic content (DNA and/or RNA) of a clinical or environmental sample is sequenced.[12] The mNGS approach is truly sequencing everything in the sample. Metagenomic approaches have allowed identification of many new viruses that were previously undiscovered.[1,11] Metagenomics has been demonstrated to be useful in human clinical diagnostics, producing a diagnosis in cases in which routine methods have failed.[11] So, if everything in the sample can be sequenced by a metagenomics approach, why use any other method for pathogen detection? Well, it is not as simple as it seems. Considering the vast majority of the nucleic acid in a clinical sample is from the host and only a very small portion is pathogen (<1%), detection of that pathogen in an overabundance of host nucleic acid is difficult, equated to finding a needle in a haystack.[12] Therefore, to increase the likelihood of detecting a pathogen or potential pathogen with a metagenomics approach, we must pretreat the sample to remove as much of the host nucleic acid as possible and/or amplify the amount of pathogen if we are to be successful[1,11]; this adds time and money. Lots of sequences (called reads) are needed with metagenomic methods to detect the pathogen, and it is important that we have adequate sequencing depth, number of repeat sequences obtained, from the pathogen to validate the detection; this also adds to the cost. In addition, metagenomics produces huge data sets that require appropriate computational resources, adequate reference databases for data analysis, and individuals with an understanding of the data produced as it relates to the clinical disease in the patient.[1,11]

Importantly, detection does not necessarily equate to pathology or causality. For example, many of the organisms detected that are associated with disease, such as bovine respiratory disease, are opportunistic pathogens. These organisms are routinely normal flora and do not cause disease unless conditions are created by other pathogens that then allow these "normal flora" to enhance the disease condition. The clinical significance of newly discovered organisms must be experimentally evaluated.[1,11] Proving an organism as a disease causative agent was traditionally done by fulfilling Koch postulates, which hinges on culturing/isolating the organism. However, considering many of the newly detected viruses or bacteria cannot be isolated, guidelines for establishing causality have been revised to exclude isolation, but the rigor for such a determination has been expanded.[11] Additionally, in considering use of NGS for veterinary diagnostics, particularly for production medicine, considerations like cost and turnaround time are significant factors that affect test use. Therefore, metagenomics at this point is still considered a research method for difficult or unusual cases rather than a routine diagnostic method.[11,12]

So, how can NGS be used as a routine diagnostic method for detection of infectious diseases in a veterinary diagnostic laboratory? Incorporation into the diagnostic laboratory must take into account cost and turnaround time, so any NGS method that reduces these has the potential to be used for routine diagnostics. One example is tNGS. What makes this different than other NGS methods is the use of targeting. For pathogens, this means incorporating capture probes specific for the pathogen to isolate it from the background genetic material or using PCR to amplify the pathogen before sequencing to increase the amount of pathogen nucleic acid in the sample above the host nucleic acid background (**Fig. 1**).[12] This process increases the

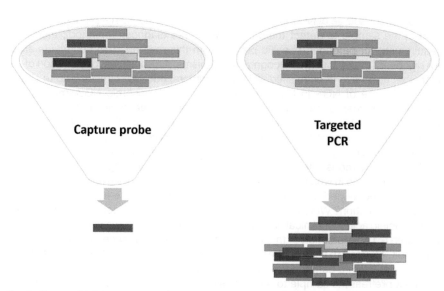

Fig. 1. Targeted NGS, capture probes versus PCR. Targeted NGS is used to target specific sequences that we want to obtain from a sample, which are present in low amounts compared with the background host nucleic acid that we do not want. We can target with capture probes to pull out those pathogens of interest from the background material or we can use PCR with primers specific for those pathogens of interest to amplify them above the background. The goal is to increase our ability to detect these pathogens that are present in very low amounts compared with the host genetic material that is present in the sample.

sensitivity of the method for pathogen detection, allowing for fewer reads needed for actionable results, as the sample has been preenriched before sequencing. With targeting by PCR, millions of needles are being added to our haystack, making detection of a needle much easier. Fewer sequencing reads generally also equates to reduced time to sequence and to analyze the data.[13] Adding additional capture probes or more primer sets specific for additional pathogens and using multiplex PCR allows us to target more pathogens in the sample.

Targeting with NGS was originally used in cancer diagnostics; whereas rare somatic mutations are difficult to detect by WGS, targeting regions with known mutations enormously increases the sensitivity to detect these genetic changes because it increases the number of reads and the sequencing depth in these regions with the mutations.[14] It has been determined that target sequencing of the key genes in the cancer genome is one of the most effective ways to identify the characteristics of the disease, and to determine treatment strategies.[14] There are multiple targeted cancer panels available in human medicine, and the majority of oncologists now use NGS results to guide cancer treatment.[15] Another targeted method is the one used for microbial detection, 16S rRNA gene NGS, and it has widespread use for evaluation of bacterial communities, such as microbiomes, entirety of organisms that colonize individual sites in the body.[12] This method is based on the capability of NGS to resolve mixed-sequence populations.[16] For example, 16S rRNA gene NGS has been commonly used to sequence the gut microbiome of multiple animal species, allowing evaluation of how different diseases, diets, supplements, and so on, affect the normal microbiome of the animal.

The drawback with targeted sequencing is that this method is limited in its ability to detect novel pathogens.[12] However, considering the targeting can be limited to known pathogens of clinical relevance, relating the results to disease pathology is not normally a daunting process with this method. With tNGS, hundreds of pathogens (including bacteria, viruses, parasites, and fungi) can be targeted with a single test; this gives tNGS an advantage over routine multiplex PCR, which is basically limited to 3 to 4 different pathogens per test, and it makes tNGS an ideal method for syndromic testing.[12,13] For example, a tNGS panel that the author's group developed for bovine testing includes 13 pathogens for bovine respiratory disease complex testing (**Box 2**).[13] The tNGS panel additionally includes pathogens associated with mastitis and reproductive disease.[13] Although NGS cannot compete with PCR with regard to speed, the sequencing data that are also provided by this method can be used to not only detect the pathogen but also characterize it.[12] The calf scours portion of the panel can detect 8 different pathogens, including viruses, parasites, and bacteria such as *Escherichia coli* and *Clostridium perfringens*, while also detecting toxins and virulence factors to confirm these are pathogenic bacterial strains.[13] For example, we can detect K99 and heat-stable and heat-labile toxins to classify an enterotoxigenic *Escherichia coli* associated with calf diarrhea directly from the fecal sample. The area of the pathogen sequenced can be leveraged to allow for variant typing or to distinguish modified live vaccine strain from wild-type strain.[13] Although a Ct value is not produced like with real-time PCR with an NGS assay, the abundance of organisms in the sample can be estimated from the number of reads that are generated that match their genomes.[13,17] More reads suggests more pathogen in the sample; however, as with any diagnostic test, the results must be interpreted in light of the patient history and clinical and pathologic findings. Detection does not always equate to disease.

Targeted Next-Generation Sequencing Workflow

There are multiple steps involved in a tNGS workflow (**Fig. 2**). This process obviously starts with appropriate sample collection and handling. As with all sequencing methods, the accuracy of NGS critically depends on the quality, integrity, and amount of the nucleic acids used from the sample. Generally, fresh frozen tissues and samples such as anticoagulated whole blood provide good-quality nucleic acids and are the best for use.[15] The sample must be representative of the clinical disease, so samples such as CSF, respiratory swabs or washes, and feces can also be used. The samples must be collected in a way to prevent nucleic acid contamination between samples. Fresh samples need to be kept refrigerated to maintain the integrity of the nucleic acid and should be sent to the laboratory as quickly as possible on ice packs (ideally using overnight shipping). One should contact one's laboratory for guidance on sample collection and transport. Once received in the laboratory, the nucleic acid must be extracted from the sample. Next, a reverse transcription step is generally run to

Box 2 Bovine respiratory disease complex syndromic testing portion of targeted next-generation sequencing panel	
Bovine viral diarrhea virus	*Mycoplasma bovis*
Infectious bovine rhinotracheitis	*Mannheimia haemolytica*
Bovine coronavirus	*Histophilus somni*
Adenovirus	*Bibersteinia trehalosi*
Parainfluenza virus	*Trueperella pyogenes*
Influenza type D	*Pasteurella multocida*
Bovine respiratory syncytial virus	

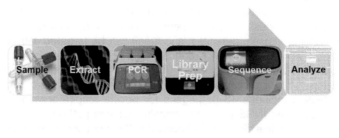

Fig. 2. Targeted NGS workflow. There are multiple steps to the targeted NGS workflow. These include obtaining the accurate clinical sample, extracting the nucleic acid from the sample, running a multiplex PCR with primers specific for infectious diseases of interest to increase the assay sensitivity, library preparation, followed by sequencing and data analysis. This is a 2- to 3-day process.

convert RNA (for RNA viruses) to DNA because DNA is required for PCR and sequencing. For our tNGS method, a multiplex PCR is performed using more than 100 pathogen-specific primers to amplify pathogens in the sample above the host background. A library preparation is then performed to prepare the sample for sequencing. For the sequencing technology the author's group uses (Ion Torrent technology, Thermo Fisher Scientific), library preparation involves an additional PCR step to add sequencing adaptors that are recognized by the machine for sequencing to occur, and if multiple samples are tested together, addition of barcode adaptors to allow separation of sequences obtained from each sample; this is typical for short read NGS technologies. Some library preparations require an enzymatic digestion or physical disruption step to create the correct-sized DNA products for sequencing. The size of the product needed depends on the sequencing platform used. For most of the sequencing platforms, the library preparation must be done manually. However, for the assay used by the author's group that uses Ion Ampliseq Technology (Thermo Fisher Scientific), they have the ability to use automated library preparation using an instrument called the Ion Chef, which significantly reduces technician hands-on time and reduces potential for human error. The library preparation has multiple steps, which makes it prone to errors. Any automation of the NGS process that is possible is beneficial to incorporation into the diagnostic laboratory for quality purposes. Sequencing with the Ion Torrent instrument is performed on a semiconductor chip. The library preparations must be loaded onto the chip. This is a long process that is performed on the Ion Chef and is run overnight in our laboratory. The sequencing part of this process actually only takes about 4 hours, but the sequencing time varies, depending on the technology used. With the Ion Torrent platform, the DNA fragments in the sample are clonally amplified on beads that are contained in wells associated with the semiconductor chip. The sequencing is done by using the DNA as the template and flowing nucleotides one at a time over the beads. Incorporation of a nucleotide into the growing strand of complementary DNA results in the release of hydrogen ions, which causes a pH change that is detected by the semiconductor chip.[15] Essentially, the sequencer is a very complex pH meter that converts the chemical change into a voltage change when a base is added and the identity of the incorporated base is known, based on which nucleotide was run over the beads.

Ion Torrent technology differs from Illumina, which is the most common sequencing technology used to date. Illumina, like Ion Torrent, also requires short reads for sequencing and uses DNA amplification for the sequencing process. Illumina calls this "sequencing by synthesis." However, instead of detecting nucleotide incorporation by release of a hydrogen bond as the DNA strand is produced, the nucleotides themselves are tagged with fluorescent markers and detection is by fluorescence. There is no chip used for Illumina sequencing, which instead uses a flow cell. Other technologies, like the Nanopore MinION, do not use DNA amplification for sequencing. The nucleic acid is sequenced directly, which in general shortens the sequencing time. For information about other sequencing technologies, see Slatko and colleagues.[4]

Once sequencing is complete, the data must be analyzed. Depending on the NGS method used, such as mNGS, this process can be very complicated and accessibility to bioinformatics expertise is very useful and potentially necessary; this requires sequence trimming to remove sequencing adaptors and barcodes, assembly of sequences, alignment of sequences to known sequences available in a database, and potentially database building to include pathogens that cause animal diseases. However, as more automated data analysis pipelines are developed and are made available, the data analysis will become more routine. Something lacking in veterinary medicine that is available in human medicine is curated databases for pathogens.[17] The sequences obtained from NGS must be aligned to a reference database for identification. The author's group generally uses the National Center for Biotechnology Information (NCBI) database for this purpose. The NCBI database contains lots of pathogen sequences, but this database is not curated, which can lead to errors when assigning pathogen classification. Using a targeted approach makes this analysis step much less complicated and allows for rapid data analysis and reporting, simply because the targeted method is limited to detection of a set of known specific pathogens and not to any and all organisms that could be present, including any that have not been previously recognized.

Based on the sheer number of steps involved, tNGS takes approximately 2 to 3 days to perform. However, turnaround time is generally longer because laboratories tend to batch samples to make the testing more cost effective. The number of reads needed for actionable results with tNGS is in the tens to hundreds of thousands, compared with millions needed for mNGS because of the low amount of relative pathogen nucleic acids in the sample. As NGS approaches become more commonplace in laboratories, and sample testing volumes increase, both testing time and cost can be reduced, potentially filling the niche currently filled by PCR-based assays.

Validation of Next-Generation Sequencing-Based Testing

Probably the biggest and most important barrier to incorporation of NGS methods for routine use in the diagnostic laboratory is validation. Diagnostic laboratories must operate under quality systems as part of their accreditation. Therefore a test must minimize variation, be able to be conducted with standard operating procedures, and must be a reproducible process, time after time, by many different people working in the laboratory. This is no small feat. Validation requires the calculation of analytical sensitivity and specificity, accuracy, precision, and limit of detection.[17] The costs to validate such large panels is tremendous if each pathogen than can be detected is validated. Also, all the different sample types that can be used have to each be validated. At present, there are no set guidelines, even in human medicine, for validation of NGS tests for pathogen detection.[17,18] As a result of time and cost, the validation work for these panels has been limited to proof of concept rather than full validation of all portions of the panel.[13,19] Regardless, the author's group has been able to incorporate validated portions of these panels into their laboratory for diagnostic use for expanded syndromic testing and are finding clinically significant organisms that would have been missed without use of the tNGS assay.[13] For example, they frequently detect *Mycoplasma bovis* from lung tissue when it was not cultured in the laboratory. If a specific PCR is not available for this organism or it is not requested, this pathogen can be easily missed because it is difficult to culture and requires special media.

SUMMARY

Although still generally considered a research tool, NGS has been incorporated into a few of the veterinary diagnostic laboratories. There are multiple ways to use the technology for infectious disease diagnostics, with metagenomics approaches providing the widest range of detection, but at the highest cost. tNGS maintains the ability to detect a huge range of pathogens but at a reduced cost compared with mNGS, making this method a viable approach for syndromic testing in the veterinary diagnostic laboratory.

CLINICS CARE POINTS

- tNGS is used for the detection of known pathogens, so this method is not for discovery of unknown organisms.
- tNGS is a molecular method similar to PCR that detects nucleic acid (DNA and RNA) from the pathogen, so the sample must be refrigerated or frozen to preserve the nucleic acid. Samples should be sent to the laboratory as soon as possible (ideally overnight on ice packs). Extremely autolyzed samples will likely not work.
- tNGS is not PCR, although it includes PCR steps. tNGS takes 2 to 3 days to perform, and results will likely take longer due to laboratory batching of samples to decrease test cost.
- tNGS is not real-time PCR. A Ct value is not obtained, but relative amounts of pathogen can be seen based on the number of reads obtained. More reads suggests more pathogen, but like any test, results must be interpreted in light of history and clinical and pathologic findings.

DISCLOSURE

The author declares no commercial or financial conflicts of interest.

REFERENCES

1. Datta S, Budhauliya R, Das B, et al. Next-generation sequencing in clinical virology: Discovery of new viruses. World J Virol 2015;4(3):265–76.
2. Besser J, Carleton HA, Gerner-Smidt P, et al. Next-generation sequencing technologies and their application to the study and control of bacterial infections. Clin Microbiol Infect 2018;24(4):335–41.
3. Preston J, VanZeeland A, Peiffer DA. Innovation at Illumina: the road to the $600 human genome. Nature Portfolio website. Available at: https://www.nature.com/articles/d42473-021-00030-9. Accessed 06/09/2022.
4. Slatko BE, Gardner AF, Ausubel FM. Overview of next-generation sequencing technologies. Curr Protoc Mol Biol 2018;122(1):e59.
5. Whole Genome Sequencing (WGS) Program. U.S. Food & Drug Administration website. 2022. Available at: https://www.fda.gov/food/science-research-food/whole-genome-sequencing-wgs-program. Accessed 06, 09, 2022.
6. Morganti S, Tarantino P, Ferraro E, et al. Next generation sequencing (NGS): a revolutionary technology in pharmacogenomics and personalized medicine in cancer. Adv Exp Med Biol 2019;1168:9–30.

7. Jacinto JGP, Häfliger IM, Borel N, et al. Clinicopathological and genomic characterization of a simmental calf with generalized bovine juvenile angiomatosis. Animals (Basel) 2021;11(3):624.

8. Ariyarathne HBPC, Correa-Luna M, Blair HT, et al. Identification of genomic regions associated with concentrations of milk fat, protein, urea and efficiency of crude protein utilization in grazing dairy cows. Genes (Basel). 2021;12(3): 456–75.

9. National animal health laboratory network antimicrobial resistance pilot project. USDA APHIS VS website. Available at: https://www.aphis.usda.gov/aphis/dashboards/tableau/amr. Accessed 06/07/2022.

10. FDA-TRACK: Progress on FDA's support of antimicrobial stewardship in veterinary settings. U.S. Food & Drug Administration website. 2022. Available at: https://www.fda.gov/about-fda/fda-track-agency-wide-program-performance/fda-track-progress-fdas-support-antimicrobial-stewardship-veterinary-settings#Antimicrobial%20Resistance. Accessed 06/07/2022.

11. Lefterova MI, Suarez CJ, Niaz B, et al. Next-generation sequencing for infectious disease diagnosis and management: a report of the association for molecular pathology. J Mol Diagn 2015;17(6):623–34.

12. Chiu CY, Miller SA. Clinical metagenomics. Nat Rev Genet 2019;20:341–55.

13. Anis E, Hawkins IK, Ilha MRS, et al. Evaluation of targeted next-generation sequencing for detection of bovine pathogens in clinical samples. J Clin Microbiol 2018;56(7):e00399-18, https://doi.org/10.1128/JCM.00399-18.

14. Nagahashi M, Shimada Y, Ichikawa H, et al. Next generation sequencing-based gene panel tests for the management of solid tumors. Cancer Sci 2019;110:6.

15. Singh RR. Next-generation sequencing in high-sensitive detection of mutations in tumors: challenges, advances, and applications. J Mol Diagn 2020;22(8): 994–1007.

16. Dulanto Chiang A, Dekker JP. From the pipeline to the bedside: advances and challenges in clinical metagenomics. J Infect Dis 2020;221(Suppl 3):S331–40.

17. Goldberg B, Sichtig H, Geyer C, et al. Making the leap from research laboratory to clinic: challenges and opportunities for next-generation sequencing in infectious disease diagnostics. mBio 2015;6(6):e01888-15.

18. Infectious disease next generation sequencing based diagnostic devices: microbial identification and detection of antimicrobial resistance and virulence markers. US Food & Drug Administration website. 2018. Available at: https://www.fda.gov/regulatory-information/search-fda-guidance-documents/infectious-disease-next-generation-sequencing-based-diagnostic-devices-microbial-identification-and. Accessed 06/09/2022.

19. Anis E, Ilha MRS, Engiles JB, et al. Evaluation of targeted next-generation sequencing for detection of equine pathogens in clinical samples. J Vet Diagn Invest 2021;33(2):227–34.

Future Directions for Ruminant Diagnostics

John Dustin Loy, DVM, PhD, DACVM[a],*, Jessie D. Monday, DVM, MS, DACVPM[b],
David R. Smith, DVM, PhD, Dipl. ACVPM, Dipl. Epidemiology[c]

KEYWORDS

- MALDI-TOF mass spectrometry • Whole genome sequencing • NGS • PCR
- Diagnostic interpretation • Diagnostic error

KEY POINTS

- Application of population-based diagnostic strategies can maximize the accuracy of diagnostic testing on herds.
- Proper sample collection, submission, and testing requests can enhance the ability to get an accurate diagnosis.
- Technological advances have resulted in tests with increased sensitivity, shortened testing time, and provide ability for broad syndromic testing.
- Interpretation of results, especially real-time PCR testing, in the face of opportunistic pathogens requires additional research to develop appropriate clinical cutoff values.
- Sensitivity of new diagnostic approaches requires additional vigilance to ensure proper linkage of detection of target nucleic acid to a clinical disease.
- Next-generation sequencing approaches provide the potential for the generation of incredible amounts of information on hosts and pathogens to stimulate new research.

INTRODUCTION

This issue of Veterinary Clinics of North America: Food Animal Practice focused on several major themes, which reviewed the application of new and emerging diagnostic technologies and approaches, the integration of these technologies with classic diagnostic methods such as culture, serology, and pathology, and population-based approaches to utilizing diagnostic information. This article will provide a forward-looking review to provide researchers, diagnosticians, specialists, and clinicians

[a] College of Veterinary Medicine, Mississippi State University, 240 Wise Center Drive, PO Box 6100, Mississippi State, MS 39762, USA; [b] Texas A&M Veterinary Medical Diagnostic Laboratory – Canyon, WT Box 60818, 3209 Russell Long Boulevard, Canyon, TX 79016, USA; [c] College of Veterinary Medicine, Mississippi State University, 240 Wise Center Drive, PO Box 6100, Mississippi State, MS 39762, USA
* Corresponding author. Nebraska Veterinary Diagnostic Center, 4040 East Campus Loop N., Lincoln, NE 68583-0907.
E-mail address: jdloy@unl.edu

Vet Clin Food Anim 39 (2023) 175–183
https://doi.org/10.1016/j.cvfa.2022.10.008
0749-0720/23/© 2022 Elsevier Inc. All rights reserved.

with some insights and perspectives to diagnostic medicine and areas that may benefit from additional research or investigation.

Applications and Interpretation of Diagnostic Testing to Individuals and Populations

The diagnostic process is one of forming beliefs about a subject's condition based on medical knowledge and information gathered about that subject, ordering diagnostic tests that might help confirm or refute those beliefs, and then using the results of those tests to modify the strength of our beliefs about the subject's condition. The process may lead to ordering additional diagnostic tests but hopefully the process ultimately leads to a diagnosis or addressing enough medical uncertainty to allow the formation of a treatment or preventive medicine action plan. The subject may be an individual or a group. New diagnostic modalities and improvements in classic techniques have made diagnostic tests even more useful as aids to gathering diagnostic data and making a diagnosis. For example, real-time PCR, whole genome sequencing (WGS), and other methods such as MALDI-TOF mass spectrometry are replacing conventional bacterial and cell culture methods and improving our ability to detect and characterize pathogens (see Loy and colleagues, "Current and Emerging Diagnostic Approaches to Bacterial Diseases of Ruminants", in this issue). However, better diagnostic tests do not relieve the veterinarian of the responsibility for gathering historical and current medical information and utilizing medical knowledge and experience to make the diagnosis. To avoid diagnostic error, the veterinarian, now and in the future, must still be a critical interpreter of diagnostic test results in the context of the clinical scenario. Unfortunately, despite the availability of better and better diagnostic tests, diagnostic error remains common in medicine.[1,2]

Diagnostic errors occur when no diagnosis is made, when actionable information is arrived at too late, or when the diagnosis or clinical assumption based in part on the diagnostic result data is wrong.[2] The problem with diagnostic error is that it may lead to inaction when action is needed or taking action that is inappropriate and potentially harmful. Sometimes, the diagnosis is correct but fails to lead to a solution. For example, a correctly identified pathogen might be an opportunist causing tissue damage and clinical signs of a disease. However, that specific pathogen might be one of several that could have taken the opportunity to invade given that the animal was unable to mount a sufficient immune response, and the immunosuppression may have been due to a variety of accumulated stressors (ie, additional component causes)[3] placed on the animal in the production system. In this case, diagnosing and correcting the system issues might be more useful than naming the pathogen.[4] To be fair, sometimes knowing the pathogen may point to the problem in the system. For example, detecting *Klebsiella pneumoniae* from a mastitis sample might appropriately lead to an investigation of the cattle's bedding as a systems-level cause of the infection. Knowing the pathogen may be useful for directing therapy, designing preventative medicine plans, or providing a prognosis. Moreover, sometimes identifying the pathogen provides critically important information, such as detecting foot and mouth disease virus or *Mycobacterium bovis*.

Diagnostic error may occur due to errors in sample collection or handling, errors inherent to a diagnostic test, errors conducting the test, or because of cognitive errors, which are errors in the thought process. The authors of Buczinski and colleagues "Interpretation and analysis of individual diagnostic tests and performance", in this issue discuss diagnostic test performance and how it is commonly communicated in terms of test sensitivity and test specificity, which reflect the likelihood of a sample from an individual with a condition to test positive, or from an individual free of the condition to test negative, respectively (see Buczinski and colleagues "Interpretation and analysis of individual diagnostic tests and performance", in this issue). Test performance is also sometimes expressed as likelihood ratios that combine information from test sensitivity and test specificity, with the likelihood of a positive result based on clinical information gathered from medical experience and examination of the situation and animal tested (see Buczinski and colleagues "Interpretation and analysis of individual diagnostic tests and performance", in this issue). The authors point out that testing as simple as auscultating for a "ping" to detect a displaced abomasum is subject to error based on the hearing ability of the veterinarian, the quality of the stethoscope, and the body condition of the cow. The size and quality of a tissue specimen or how it is handled before it gets to the laboratory may interfere with accurate test results, as can the stage of the disease process at the time of sampling. Cognitive errors may be due to lack of knowledge, which may be on the part of the individual and that individual's experience, or may be due to lack of scientific knowledge in the general medical and diagnostic fields. Sometimes, cognitive error occurs because we fail to correctly estimate the likelihood of a condition.[5] We may fail to consider the condition or we overestimate or underestimate its likelihood. If we fail to consider a condition, we may not consider running diagnostic tests that could aid the diagnosis. If we fail to accurately estimate the likelihood of the condition (eg, fail to accurately estimate pretest probability), then we might not correctly interpret the results of a diagnostic test, or we may order tests that we should have known were going to be misleading (see Buczinski article). The ability to accurately estimate pretest probability is a critical skill of diagnostic test interpretation and therefore an important component of veterinary education. The authors of Buczinski and colleagues "Interpretation and analysis of individual diagnostic tests and performance", in this serial explain how to use pretest probability and diagnostic test performance to estimate how likely a positive or negative test result reflects the true condition of the animal. Any test result, positive or negative, has a likelihood of being correct, ranging from 0 to 100%, depending on the clinical circumstances which must be evaluated through a lens of clinical judgement (ie, to form prior beliefs or pretest probability). Therefore, for now and well into the future, the strategy of sending samples to the laboratory to test for anything and everything, and letting the laboratory make the clinical diagnosis in the absence of clinical judgement, risks failure. No test can reliably provide enough information to supplant the need for a disease risk assessment based on history, patient evaluation, and veterinary critical thinking skills in the diagnostic process.

We also learn in Buczinski and colleagues "Interpretation and analysis of individual diagnostic tests and performance", of this issue that sometimes a single diagnostic test may fall short of the goal of aiding a diagnosis (see Buczinski and colleagues). This may be because in some circumstances either a positive test result or a negative test result is unlikely to reflect the true condition of animal. In these circumstances, it may be useful to strategically use more than one test to help rule in or rule out a diagnosis. The veterinarian must know what strategy of multiple testing to use. Serial testing helps to improve overall test specificity at some cost to test sensitivity. Serial testing is often a useful strategy when the condition is rare or unlikely and the concern is about poor positive predictive value. This is a common scenario when screening healthy appearing animals for a health condition or contagious disease. Parallel testing helps to improve overall test sensitivity at the cost of test specificity. Parallel testing is often useful when a condition is likely, and the concern is about poor negative predictive value. Sometimes, our prior beliefs about an animal's condition are strong enough that a test result either simply confirms our expectation or is likely to be wrong in the case it does not match our pretest clinical suspicion. In those situations, there is very little utility in running the test if definitive clinical diagnosis is the only goal of testing.

The diagnosis of a condition in an individual animal often has implications for the herd. Because ruminant animals are often managed as herd animals, we may (rightly or wrongly) assign a problem diagnosed (rightly or wrongly) in an individual to the group. For example, if we diagnose Johne disease in an individual animal, we will likely assume that *Mycobacterium avium* spp. paratuberculosis is being transmitted among others in the herd. It is now a "Johne's herd" with important economic consequences associated with that designation. Therefore, an incorrect diagnosis in an individual may be even more consequential at the herd level. The possibility of a herd-level misdiagnosis becomes greater when testing multiple animals. The problem of misclassifying a herd by a health condition is more often a problem of test specificity than test sensitivity. Herd-level sensitivity increases as more animals are tested because the possibility of a false-negative herd-level classification decreases as more animals are tested. However, the possibility of a false herd-level classification increases as more animals are tested because there is a greater opportunity to detect a false-positive testing individual.[6]

In Elizabeth Parkers, "Diagnostic strategies for ruminant populations", in this issue, Dr Parker describes the many reasons a veterinarian might want to test multiple animals within a herd. For example, one may wish to know if a pathogen or disease condition is present at all in a herd, for example, to evaluate biosecurity. Otherwise, one may want to know how prevalent a pathogen or health condition is in a population, for example, to evaluate biocontainment. Moreover, one may want to know if an intervention had an effect on the prevalence of a pathogen or condition in a population. Dr Parker provides formulas for calculating the number of animals to test for various purposes including in situations where the sampling strategy is complex, such as in clustered sampling. Similar in concept to how the quality of the sample may affect the results of testing an individual, so too does the number of animals and their likelihood to have the condition of interest affect the reliability of testing within populations.

Veterinarians are hindered from following the advice in this issue for improving their skills at diagnostic interpretation because they often cannot find accurate information about test performance, information to aid estimates of pretest probability, and because the causes of many conditions we observe in animals are poorly studied systems effects or are not yet known to science. Therefore, in addition to developing new test modalities, an important focus of future veterinary research must be on evaluation of the performance of diagnostic tests on clinically relevant samples, typically in the absence of a gold-standard reference tests; more field studies to better understand the frequency of the occurrence of health conditions. In addition, for population-level investigations, future research is needed to help inform veterinarians about expected within and between herd prevalence in various relevant scenarios and the expected intracluster correlation. Finally, research is needed to aid understanding what factors in the production system modify the frequency of health conditions; and we need to better understand the microscopic and macroscopic factors that cause undesirable health outcomes.

Integration of Emerging Technologies with Classic Diagnostics

Diagnostic testing has traditionally relied on classic methods and approaches, many of which are gold standard, or the best test to assess the true disease status. These methods provide the foundation for what is known and understood about animal diseases and, thus, are heavily integrated into how veterinarians use testing as part of their diagnostic strategies. Many of these methods remain critically important to veterinary diagnostic laboratories (VDLs) and testing laboratories. Clinical pathology, anatomical and histopathology, antimicrobial susceptibility, and serological testing have all been mainstays of VDL diagnostic testing for decades and remain critically important to veterinarians. Research continues to build on how to apply these methods, both existing tests and newly developed, to disease diagnosis and prevention in ruminants.

Clinical pathology testing has long been established as quick and reliable modes of diagnostic investigation. Evaluation of individual animal tissues, blood, and/or fluids has the potential to provide valuable information on current immune, physiologic, and cytologic statuses. In "Submitting High-Quality Clinical Pathology Samples for Best Results" Author Wikander discusses the limitations of clinical pathology testing and interpretation based on sample acquisition and handling. The samples provided for testing and clinical pathologist evaluation must be representative of the current disorder under diagnostic investigation and of quality to allow for proper evaluation. Dr Wikander discusses test selection based on patient assessment as well as sample collection based on desired clinical pathology testing. Clinical pathology testing options are no longer limited to sending samples to referral laboratories. Many clinics have bench top and chute side testing options. The ability of these point of care diagnostic options to provide accurate and reliable data continues to increase. Some in-house equipment options now have ruminant specific analytes with ruminant species-specific reference intervals. Accurate and reliable results from in-house equipment require a quality assurance program. Dr Wikander reviews the options for clinics to develop protocols for equipment maintenance, calibration, and quality control monitoring. Digital cytology evaluation options also exist with some referral and private laboratories that allow for pictures of tissue cytology slides to be sent for evaluation by clinical pathologists with results provided in hours, rather than the days needed when slides must be sent into referral laboratories. The use of digital cytology programs should continue to increase and improve as image technology and clinical staff experience in providing quality digital images for evaluation increases.

Metabolic profiling is an option for utilizing clinical pathology techniques at the herd level to investigate population-level disease risks and nutritional status. Dr Van Saun discusses proper metabolic profiling testing plans and the strengths and limitations of this population based testing in Robert J. Van Sauns "Metabolic Profiling in Ruminant Diagnostics" in this issue. As with individual animal clinical pathology testing, diagnostic success depends on proper sample collection and handling. Interpretation of the findings, as well as the format of the results reported, depend on the goal of the testing and proper selection of animals included in each tested group or population. The concept of metabolic profile testing to address animal performance, health, or reproductive issues associated with metabolic changes occurring during the transition period has evolved since introduction in the 1970s.[7] Dr Van Saun reviews diagnostic rationales for metabolic profiling, including the development of the initial diagnostic hypothesis, and summarizes the current blood analytes available that may meet the diagnostic needs of those utilizing metabolic profiling to investigate or monitor populations. Robert J. Van Sauns "Metabolic Profiling in Ruminant Diagnostics" in this issue concludes with a brief discussion on potential future applications of metabolic profiling using milk rather than serum samples and other technologies that would allow for point of care on-farm testing.

Anatomical pathology and histopathology remain a critical leg to the stool of veterinary diagnostic testing. Histopathology is essential for the diagnosis of many diseases, some of which can only be diagnosed with this modality. However, optimal utility of the diagnostic strengths of histopathology requires the pathologist has an adequate clinical history, has properly collected and fixed samples, and has an understanding of the relationship of the observed histopathology to any gross pathology present. In "Anatomical Pathology/Histopathology for Diagnostics" Hille and colleagues review the fundamentals of tissue sampling, fixation and provide an overview of applications to several specific ruminant diseases, and include specific tissues that are critical to submit for evaluation for these diseases. One important discussion in this review is how pathological findings can help practitioners not only look at potential causality but may also assist in determining temporality. The authors describe situations where disease may seem acute clinically but on histopathological examination chronic and more long-term lesions were viewed. This information would be more helpful in determining the underlying cause and potential treatment and prevention strategies in the future.

Antimicrobial susceptibility testing remains a critical service provided by VDLs, which helps practitioners provide data-driven recommendations on prudent antimicrobial usage. In "Application and Interpretation of Antimicrobial Susceptibility Testing" Fajt and Lubbers review the application and interpretation of AST, including a when and how to use this testing in a variety of scenarios. Importantly, included are some guidelines on how breakpoints might be applied to minor species such as sheep and goats, what to do when you have an MIC in the absence of a clinical breakpoint, and how published data on AST might be applied to empirical decision making. One important consideration the authors make is in regards to application of genomic technologies to examining AST and the limitations thereof. The lack of clinical validation for genomic approaches to AST is a pitfall to be recognized and as both genomic and AST technologies advance, future research may enable these to be further developed and new tools validated for clinical use may be possible.

Another area where technology has significantly improved the testing process is in the area of serology. In "SEROLOGY IN BOVINE INFECTIOUS DISEASE DIAGNOSIS" Dr Woolums reviews the types and application of serological testing available for ruminant practitioners. Although its development dates back to the early 1970s, the enzyme-linked immunosorbent assay (ELISA), and variations of this approach, has revolutionized diagnostic testing.[8,9] Variations of this original assay format have enabled the detection of antibodies, detection of antigens, and enabled developments of variations such as competitive ELISA that are extremely sensitive, and rapid lateral flow assays for a number of veterinary diseases that are rapid and can be used in the field.[10] The ELISA-based assay formats are typically simple, can be automated, and have excellent diagnostic performance and when combined with a reader deliver quantifiable results, all of which support their widespread use (see Woolums). Although getting a test result from many of these tests is often straightforward, interpretation can be challenging. Dr Woolums reminds us that interpretation of results requires information on if the agent is suspected to cause transient versus life-long infections, vaccination history, and potential for maternal antibodies. Additionally, the importance of paired serum samples to determine if there are rising antibody levels is highlighted as a useful way to assist interpretation.

New and Emerging Diagnostic Technologies

The application of new technologies to veterinary diagnostic testing has provided the ability to generate tremendous amounts of information from even a single sample. As reviewed by Dr Wilkes in "Next Generation Approaches for Diagnostics," these technologies include next-generation sequencing (NGS)-based approaches that can be used in several diagnostic applications, such as screening for large numbers of known diseases and agents, as well as novel pathogen discovery. NGS-based approaches also enable whole genome sequences (WGS) of pathogen isolates and strains to be generated. Dr Wilkes describes one recently developed example using targeted NGS for bovine pathogens, which can be integrated into diagnostic laboratory work-flows.[11] Integration of targeted NGS in diagnostic laboratories would enable screening for tremendous numbers of pathogens, and have the potential to reduce per test cost, as well as, testing and analysis time in VDLs. Further improvements in sequencing technologies, data analysis workflows, and clinical validation are needed before such methods become widespread in diagnostics; however, these gaps are rapidly closing, and we may see a future where NGS provides a holistic diagnostic approach to infectious diseases and beyond.[12] In addition to individual diagnostic testing, these approaches are rapidly being applied at the population level through human public health infrastructures, and such tools could readily be applied to veterinary pathogens in a similar manner.[13]

Other new advances include applications of mass analytical instruments, such as MALDI-TOF, once only found in a chemical or toxicology laboratory. The data generated from these instruments can be leveraged into powerful tools for microbial identification and typing.[14] In Loy and colleagues, the authors review how this method has revolutionized a VDL's ability to rapidly identify and type pathogens isolated from diagnostic samples. For example, to identify *Salmonella* in a fecal culture by classic approaches took several passages through selective and nonselective media, biochemical tests, and screening with specific antiserum. Those same suspect colonies now can be identified using MALDI-TOF in minutes. Additionally, identification no longer depends on biochemical based-testing, which has greatly improved the ability to identify challenging groups, such as anaerobic and fastidious bacteria.

Synergistic approaches using new diagnostic technologies such as NGS and MALDI-TOF have resulted in new diagnostic tests. For example, using NGS approaches to WGS of bacterial genomes has allowed for the identification of variants, distinct genotypes, potential virulence factors, and antimicrobial resistance genes. Mass spectrum from sequenced strains can then be entered into MALDI-TOF databases or used with bioinformatics and machine learning classifier tools to develop genotyping assays. However, both WGS and MALDI-TOF–based typing approaches are only as strong as the metadata associated with the strains, which primarily come from diagnostic submission information. These data are key to determining which strains are most likely associated with disease. Another gap is the bias toward diagnostics, where there is a paucity of strains that originate from normal healthy animals for comparison. Future studies on WGS of pathogens will require robust metadata and clinical and geographic information, where possible, to enable additional experimental studies. These approaches are especially critical to further the field's understanding of opportunistic pathogens, where a wide range of potential pathogenicity and diverse genetics is likely to be circulating in animal populations.

Application of NGS and other sequencing technologies have also allowed for novel pathogen discovery. Viruses have recently been found associated with diseases that include Parechoviruses, influenza viruses, and others in ruminants.[15,16] As reviewed by Dr Wang in "Diagnostics for viral pathogens in veterinary diagnostic laboratories", in this issue, these technologies are also being studied to identify emerging variants such as those in bovine coronaviruses or pestiviruses. Several examples of emerging diseases in swine are provided to show how genomic sequencing tools may be applied to these emerging pathogens. Additionally, the authors in this section remind us of the importance of the temporal nature of viral infections. Diagnosis of these infections using virus detection depends on multiple factors but timing is especially important because the window is much smaller. Additionally, the widespread use of modified live vaccines also provides some challenges in interpretation of virus detection, especially at low levels, and can be difficult to distinguish from early or late infections, or nonoptimal sample types.

SUMMARY

In spite of advanced diagnostic technology, the concepts for improving individual and herd-level diagnostic test interpretation will remain important to making an accurate diagnosis well into the future. The requirement for high quality, relevant, and appropriate samples remains critical to achieving diagnostic success, regardless of the testing method. New technologies are rapidly enhancing the sensitivity and power of diagnostic testing but this has complicated analysis, interpretation, and comparison with classic diagnostic approaches. However, regardless of the method, testing fundamentals remain the same, and results should be interpreted in the context of a complete and through clinical picture and used to inform treatment and prevention plans.

CLINICS CARE POINTS

- Assessment of pretest probability and diagnostic test performance are a critical part of achieving an accurate diagnosis from a test result.
- Herd-level testing can be complex in both sample strategies and interpretation and requires a clear understanding of the testing objectives.
- Histopathology and clinical pathology are extremely useful for diagnostics but require proper sample collection, handling, and clinical history.
- New technologies such as next-generation sequencing and MALDI-TOF have revolutionized the amounts and types of information that can be generated from diagnostic samples but still require appropriate metadata and clinical history for interpretation.

ACKNOWLEDGMENTS

This work is a contribution of the Nebraska Veterinary Diagnostic Center (Loy), the Texas A&M Veterinary Medical Diagnostic Laboratory - Veterinary Services (Monday), and the Beef Cattle Population Health and Reproduction Program at Mississippi State University (Smith) The authors' would like to acknowledge the support of the staff, faculty, and students of their respective institutions.

DISCLOSURE

This work (Smith) is supported by the Agriculture and Food Research Initiative Competitive Grants Program grant no. 2018-69003-28706 from the USDA National Institute of Food and Agriculture. Any opinions, findings, conclusions, or recommendations expressed in this publication are those of the authors and do not necessarily reflect the view of the U.S. Department of Agriculture.

REFERENCES

1. Graber ML. The incidence of diagnostic error in medicine. BMJ Qual Saf 2013; 22(Suppl 2):ii21–7.
2. Sheikh A, Donaldson L, Dhingra-Kumar N, et al. Diagnostic Errors: Technical Series on Safer Primary Care. Geneva: World Health Organization; 2016.

3. Rothman KJ. Causes. Am J Epidemiol 1976;104:587–92. In File.
4. Smith DR, Wills RW, Woodruff KA. Epidemiology's adoption of system dynamics is a natural extension of population thinking. Vet Clin North Am Food Anim Pract Jul 2022;38(2):245–59.
5. McGee D. Cognitive errors in clinical decision making. 2018. Available at: https://www.merckmanuals.com/professional/special-subjects/clinical-decision-making/cognitive-errors-in-clinical-decision-making. Accessed August 25, 2018.
6. Smith DR. Epidemiologic tools for biosecurity and biocontainment. Vet Clin North Am Food Anim Pract 2002;18(1):157–75.
7. Payne JM, Dew SM, Manston R, et al. The use of a metabolic profile test in dairy herds. Vet Rec 1970;87(6):150–8.
8. Van Weemen BK, Schuurs A. Immunoassay using antigen—enzyme conjugates. FEBS Lett 1971;15(3):232–6.
9. Engvall E, Perlmann P. Enzyme-linked immunosorbent assay (ELISA) quantitative assay of immunoglobulin G. Immunochemistry. 1971;8(9):871–4.
10. O'Connor TP, Lawrence J, Andersen P, et al. Chapter 8.1 - immunoassay applications in veterinary diagnostics. In: Wild D, editor. The immunoassay handbook. Fourth Edition. Elsevier; 2013. p. 623–45.
11. Anis E, Hawkins Ian K, Ilha Marcia RS, et al. Evaluation of targeted next-generation sequencing for detection of bovine pathogens in clinical samples. J Clin Microbiol 2018;56(7). 003999-e418.
12. Eloit M, Iecuit m. The diagnosis of infectious diseases by whole genome next generation sequencing: a new era is opening. Opinion. Front Cell Infect Microbiol 2014. https://doi.org/10.3389/fcimb.2014.00025.
13. Gwinn M, MacCannell D, Armstrong GL. Next-generation sequencing of infectious pathogens. JAMA 2019;321(9):893–4.
14. Seng P, Drancourt M, Gouriet F, et al. Ongoing revolution in bacteriology: routine identification of bacteria by matrix-assisted laser desorption ionization time-of-flight mass spectrometry. Clin Infect Dis 2009;49(4):543–51. https://doi.org/10.1086/600885.
15. Oba M, Sakaguchi S, Wu H, et al. First isolation and genomic characterization of bovine parechovirus from faecal samples of cattle in Japan. J Gen Virol 2022; 103(2). https://doi.org/10.1099/jgv.0.001718.
16. Hause Ben M, Collin Emily A, Liu R, et al. Characterization of a novel influenza virus in cattle and swine: proposal for a new genus in the orthomyxoviridae family. mBio 2014;5(2). 000311-e114.

Moving?

Make sure your subscription moves with you!

To notify us of your new address, find your **Clinics Account Number** (located on your mailing label above your name), and contact customer service at:

Email: journalscustomerservice-usa@elsevier.com

800-654-2452 (subscribers in the U.S. & Canada)
314-447-8871 (subscribers outside of the U.S. & Canada)

Fax number: 314-447-8029

Elsevier Health Sciences Division
Subscription Customer Service
3251 Riverport Lane
Maryland Heights, MO 63043

*To ensure uninterrupted delivery of your subscription, please notify us at least 4 weeks in advance of move.

ELSEVIER

9780323938372